Novel Methods of Diagnostics of Thyroid and Parathyroid Lesions

Novel Methods of Diagnostics of Thyroid and Parathyroid Lesions

Editors

Marek Ruchala
Ewelina Szczepanek-Parulska

MDPI • Basel • Beijing • Wuhan • Barcelona • Belgrade • Manchester • Tokyo • Cluj • Tianjin

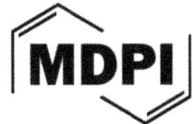

Editors
Marek Ruchala
Poznan University of Medical Sciences
Poland

Ewelina Szczepanek-Parulska
Poznan University of Medical Sciences
Poland

Editorial Office
MDPI
St. Alban-Anlage 66
4052 Basel, Switzerland

This is a reprint of articles from the Special Issue published online in the open access journal *Journal of Clinical Medicine* (ISSN 2077-0383) (available at: https://www.mdpi.com/journal/jcm/special_issues/Thyroid_Nodules).

For citation purposes, cite each article independently as indicated on the article page online and as indicated below:

LastName, A.A.; LastName, B.B.; LastName, C.C. Article Title. *Journal Name* **Year**, *Volume Number*, Page Range.

ISBN 978-3-0365-4993-4 (Hbk)
ISBN 978-3-0365-4994-1 (PDF)

© 2022 by the authors. Articles in this book are Open Access and distributed under the Creative Commons Attribution (CC BY) license, which allows users to download, copy and build upon published articles, as long as the author and publisher are properly credited, which ensures maximum dissemination and a wider impact of our publications.

The book as a whole is distributed by MDPI under the terms and conditions of the Creative Commons license CC BY-NC-ND.

Contents

About the Editors vii

Ewelina Szczepanek-Parulska and Marek Ruchala
Editorial on the Special Issue "Novel Methods of Diagnostics of Thyroid and Parathyroid Lesions"
Reprinted from: *J. Clin. Med.* **2022**, *11*, 932, doi:10.3390/jcm11040932 1

Laura Guglielmetti, Sina Schmidt, Mirjam Busch, Joachim Wagner, Ali Naddaf, Barbara Leitner, Simone Harsch, Andreas Zielke and Constantin Smaxwil
How Long Does It Take to Regain Normocalcaemia in the Event of Postsurgical Hypoparathyroidism? A Detailed Time Course Analysis
Reprinted from: *J. Clin. Med.* **2022**, *11*, 3202, doi:10.3390/jcm11113202 7

Constantin Smaxwil, Philip Aschoff, Gerald Reischl, Mirjam Busch, Joachim Wagner, Julia Altmeier, Oswald Ploner and Andreas Zielke
[^{18}F]fluoro-ethylcholine-PET Plus 4D-CT (FEC-PET-CT): A Break-Through Tool to Localize the "Negative" Parathyroid Adenoma. One Year Follow Up Results Involving 170 Patients
Reprinted from: *J. Clin. Med.* **2021**, *10*, 1648, doi:10.3390/jcm10081648 21

Constantin Smaxwil, Miriam Aleker, Julia Altmeier, Ali Naddaf, Mirjam Busch, Joachim Wagner, Simone Harsch, Oswald Ploner and Andreas Zielke
Neuromonitoring of the Recurrent Laryngeal Nerve Reduces the Rate of Bilateral Vocal Cord Dysfunction in Planned Bilateral Thyroid Procedures
Reprinted from: *J. Clin. Med.* **2021**, *10*, 740, doi:10.3390/jcm10040740 33

Chien-Ling Hung, Yu-Chen Hsu, Shih-Ming Huang and Chung-Jye Hung
Application of Tissue Aspirate Parathyroid Hormone Assay for Imaging Suspicious Neck Lesions in Patients with Complicated Recurrent or Persistent Renal Hyperparathyroidism
Reprinted from: *J. Clin. Med.* **2021**, *10*, 329, doi:10.3390/jcm10020329 43

Zbigniew Adamczewski, Magdalena Stasiak, Bartłomiej Stasiak, Magdalena Adamczewska and Andrzej Lewiński
Interobserver Agreement and Plane-Dependent Intraobserver Variability of Shear Wave Sonoelastography in the Differential Diagnosis of Ectopic Thymus Tissue
Reprinted from: *J. Clin. Med.* **2021**, *10*, 214, doi:10.3390/jcm10020214 53

Magdalena Stasiak, Zbigniew Adamczewski, Renata Stawerska, Bartłomiej Stasiak and Andrzej Lewiński
Application of Shear Wave Sonoelastography in the Differential Diagnosis of Extra- and Intra-Thyroidal Ectopic Thymic Tissue
Reprinted from: *J. Clin. Med.* **2020**, *9*, 3816, doi:10.3390/jcm9123816 65

Jacek Gawrychowski, Grzegorz J. Kowalski, Grzegorz Buła, Adam Bednarczyk, Dominika Żadło, Zbigniew Niedzielski, Agata Gawrychowska and Henryk Koziołek
Surgical Management of Primary Hyperparathyroidism—Clinicopathologic Study of 1019 Cases from a Single Institution
Reprinted from: *J. Clin. Med.* **2020**, *9*, 3540, doi:10.3390/jcm9113540 77

Katarzyna Wieczorek-Szukala, Janusz Kopczynski, Aldona Kowalska and Andrzej Lewinski
Snail-1 Overexpression Correlates with Metastatic Phenotype in BRAF^{V600E} Positive Papillary Thyroid Carcinoma
Reprinted from: *J. Clin. Med.* **2020**, *9*, 2701, doi:10.3390/jcm9092701 87

Ewelina Szczepanek-Parulska, Kosma Wolinski, Katarzyna Dobruch-Sobczak, Patrycja Antosik, Anna Ostalowska, Agnieszka Krauze, Bartosz Migda, Agnieszka Zylka, Malgorzata Lange-Ratajczak, Tomasz Banasiewicz, Marek Dedecjus, Zbigniew Adamczewski, Rafal Z. Slapa, Robert K. Mlosek, Andrzej Lewinski and Marek Ruchala
S-Detect Software vs. EU-TIRADS Classification: A Dual-Center Validation of Diagnostic Performance in Differentiation of Thyroid Nodules
Reprinted from: *J. Clin. Med.* **2020**, *9*, 2495, doi:10.3390/jcm9082495 . . . . **99**

Kirk Jensen, Shilpa Thakur, Aneeta Patel, Maria Cecilia Mendonca-Torres, John Costello, Cristiane Jeyce Gomes-Lima, Mary Walter, Leonard Wartofsky, Kenneth Dale Burman, Athanasios Bikas, Dorina Ylli, Vasyl V. Vasko and Joanna Klubo-Gwiezdzinska
Detection of BRAFV600E in Liquid Biopsy from Patients with Papillary Thyroid Cancer Is Associated with Tumor Aggressiveness and Response to Therapy
Reprinted from: *J. Clin. Med.* **2020**, *9*, 2481, doi:10.3390/jcm9082481 . . . . **113**

Solène Castellnou, Jean-Christophe Lifante, Stéphanie Polazzi, Léa Pascal, Françoise Borson-Chazot and Antoine Duclos
Influence of Care Pathway on Thyroid Nodule Surgery Relevance: A Historical Cohort Study
Reprinted from: *J. Clin. Med.* **2020**, *9*, 2271, doi:10.3390/jcm9072271 . . . . **127**

About the Editors

Marek Ruchala

Marek Ruchala graduated from Poznan University of Medical Sciences in 1988 and has worked in the Department of Endocrinology, Metabolism and Internal Medicine since then. He received his PhD degree in 1997, became an associate professor in 2008 and professor of medicine in 2011. Since 2011, he has been the head of the Department of Endocrinology, Metabolism and Internal Medicine. He is a specialist in internal medicine, endocrinology and nuclear medicine. His scientific and clinical activity is focused, but not limited to, thyroid diseases (especially thyroid developmental abnormalities, thyroid nodular disease, thyroid cancer, thyroiditis and novel techniques of thyroid imaging). He is a former or present member of the editorial board or guest editor of many scientific journals, e.g., *Journal of Clinical Endocrinology and Metabolism, Frontiers in Endocrinology, Endokrynologia Polska, Oncoreview, Thyroid Research, Nuclear Medicine Review*, and *Journal of Clinical Medicine*. He is an author or co-author of about 885 publications and congress communications at national or international levels (total impact factor of 783.769). He has been cited 3239 times (2724 without self-citations); his Hirsch index is equal to 27. He is an active member of scientific organisations. In 2016–2021, he was the President of Polish Society of Endocrinology and delegate of European Society of Endocrinology Council of Affiliated Societies (ECAS). Since 2021, he has been the past President and board member of the Polish Society of Endocrinology. Since 2015, he has been a chairman of the Medical Sciences Committee of the of Poznan branch of Polish Academy of Sciences. In 2016, he has become the Rector's Plenipotentiary for the Heliodor Święcicki Clinical Hospital in Poznań. Since 2017, he has been the secretary of Polish Thyroid Association and a member of the Central Commission for Scientific Degrees and Titles for 2 017–2020. In 2019, he was elected to the position of the Chancellor for Science of the Poznan University of Medical Sciences. He has been repeatedly awarded for his scientific, didactic and organizational achievements, e.g., by the Rector of Poznan University of Medical Sciences, Polish Academy of Arts and Science, and the Minister of Health. In 2014, he was awarded the 1st Degree Prize Władysław Biegański for outstanding didactic and educational achievements at the Poznan University of Medical Sciences. He has over 30 years of experience in thyroid ultrasound examination and fine-needle aspiration biopsy. He leads courses and workshops for medical doctors on thyroid ultrasound examination and biopsy.

Ewelina Szczepanek-Parulska

Ewelina Szczepanek-Parulska graduated from Poznan University of Medical Sciences in 2008. In 2010, she received her PhD and became an assistant professor in 2015 and a professor of medicine in 2019. She is a specialist in internal medicine and endocrinology. She works in the Department of Endocrinology, Metabolism and Internal Medicine of Poznan University of Medical Sciences, where she works on the clinical ward, endocrine outpatient clinic and holds a position as the head of the department of ultrasound diagnostics of endocrine glands. Both her scientific and clinical activities are focused on thyroid diseases, especially thyroid developmental abnormalities, thyroid nodular disease, thyroid cancer, thyroiditis and novel techniques of thyroid imaging. She has over 10 years of experience in thyroid ultrasound examination and biopsy. She is a lecturer of courses and workshops on thyroid ultrasound and biopsy for students and medical doctors. She is an author or co-author of about 290 publications and congress communications at the national and international levels (total Impact Factor 288.117). She has been cited 1066 times (898 without self-citations); her Hirsch index is equal to 19. For her scientific and didactic activity, she has been awarded by the Polish Society of Endocrinology, the Rector of Poznan University of Medical Sciences, the President of Poznan, the Polish Minister of Health as well as the Polish Academy of Arts and Science. She is an active member of scientific organisations. From 2012 to 2016, she was president of the section of young endocrinologists of the Polish Society of Endocrinology (Club 30) and a secretary of the Greater Poland branch of the Polish Thyroid Association. Since 2016, she has been president of the section of ultrasonography of Polish Society of Endocrinology. From 2016 to 2021, she was a board member of Greater Poland branch of Polish Society of Endocrinology. Since 2021 she has become a vice-president of Greater Poland branch of the Polish Society of Endocrinology. She is a former or present member of the editorial boards or served as a guest editor of many scientific journals, e.g., the *Journal of Clinical Medicine, Frontiers in Endocrinology, Endokrynologia Polska, BMC Endocrine Disorders*, and the *Journal of Ultrasonography*.

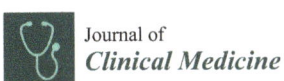

Editorial

Editorial on the Special Issue "Novel Methods of Diagnostics of Thyroid and Parathyroid Lesions"

Ewelina Szczepanek-Parulska * and Marek Ruchala

Department of Endocrinology, Metabolism and Internal Medicine, Poznan University of Medical Sciences, 61-701 Poznan, Poland; mruchala@ump.edu.pl
* Correspondence: ewelinaparulska@gmail.com

Thyroid nodular disease is one of the most frequent endocrine diseases. The prevalence of thyroid focal lesions detected by imaging techniques according to studies on different populations ranges from 10 to 70% [1,2]. In a population of women over 50 years of age, approximately half of them would have a thyroid focal lesion. This, in turn, poses an important diagnostic dilemma, as only the minority (3–15%) of such lesions exhibit malignancy [3]. The standard investigations of the thyroid nodules consist of ultrasonography coupled with qualification of the lesions for cytological examination. The pivotal role of ultrasound examination is to estimate the risk of malignancy and to select lesions for a fine-needle aspiration biopsy (FNAB). The results of cytological assessment directly determine the decision regarding the treatment. Unfortunately, both conventional ultrasonography and biopsy have certain limitations. Moreover, the evaluation of an increasing number of thyroid incidentalomas constitutes a huge burden on the healthcare system. The performance of conventional ultrasound in the differentiation of thyroid nodules is moderate, with a sensitivity equal to 68–100% and specificity ranging within 67–94%. It must be followed by a FNAB—an invasive procedure yielding inconclusive results in approximately 15–30% (3/4 of them will eventually prove to be benign on histopathology). In 2015 >600,000 of FNABs were performed in the USA [4]. Hence, there is a need for a non-invasive technique which would help to reliably assess the thyroid nodules malignancy risk. High hopes have been pinned on sonoelastography and the application of artificial intelligence [5]. In addition, molecular studies have become an increasingly useful and available tool in thyroid cancer risk assessment [6,7]. In particular, we hope that the introduction of these methods will allow us to reduce the amount of invasive practices performed unnecessarily in patients with benign nodules. It is also very important to evaluate whether the actual clinical practice guidelines are followed and how this influences the proper qualification of patients for thyroidectomy [8]. On the other hand, the techniques of surgical management are being constantly improved (mini-invasive procedures, monitoring of laryngeal nerve), which contributes to better outcomes, reduces the number of complications, and results in better post-surgery quality of life for the patients [9].

Another frequent endocrine disease that poses both a diagnostic and therapeutic challenge is primary hyperparathyroidism (PHP) [10–12]. It is diagnosed most frequently in women during the perimenopausal age, while male patients are affected four times less frequently [13]. However, when the underlying genetic cause such as MEN syndrome is present, PHP might also be diagnosed much earlier in life [14]. The incidence in the USA is approximated at 0.86% of the population [15], while the estimations for normocalcemic hyperparathyroidism vary widely according to different studies, and ranges from 0.4 to 11%; however, some of those cases are supposed to be related to vitamin D deficiency as opposed to classical PHP. Nevertheless, it is obvious that in developed countries, the diagnostic rate of PHP has increased over the past several decades. Better access to both biochemical evaluation and imaging diagnostics might contribute to that fact [13]. Better recognition of PHP is related to better diagnostics of localisation of the primary lesion, which improves the outcomes and enables a mini-invasive approach during parathyroidectomy.

Citation: Szczepanek-Parulska, E.; Ruchala, M. Editorial on the Special Issue "Novel Methods of Diagnostics of Thyroid and Parathyroid Lesions". *J. Clin. Med.* **2022**, *11*, 932. https://doi.org/10.3390/jcm11040932

Received: 17 January 2022
Accepted: 9 February 2022
Published: 11 February 2022

Publisher's Note: MDPI stays neutral with regard to jurisdictional claims in published maps and institutional affiliations.

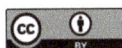

Copyright: © 2022 by the authors. Licensee MDPI, Basel, Switzerland. This article is an open access article distributed under the terms and conditions of the Creative Commons Attribution (CC BY) license (https://creativecommons.org/licenses/by/4.0/).

The aim of this review is to present the current challenges and novel methods of diagnostics and management of thyroid nodular disease and PHP, with a particular emphasis on the issues described in the papers from the Special Issue entitled "Novel Methods of Diagnostics of Thyroid and Parathyroid Lesions", published by the *Journal of Clinical Medicine*.

In the study by Adamczewski et al., a possible impact of the probe plane (longitudinal vs. transverse) on the elasticity values measured by ShearWave Elastography (SWE) method was evaluated [16]. In the study, the SWE technique was shown to present high intra- and interobserver agreement for the measurement of elastic properties of ectopic thymus (ET) and surrounding thyroid parenchyma. Important statistical differences were noted between obtained elasticity values, but not for relative elasticity scores. The authors explained this phenomenon by possible anisotropy-related artifacts; however, they also stated that the observed differences do not significantly affect the reliability of the method. The authors concluded that awareness of the existence of plane-dependent differences is crucial for proper interpretation of the measured values.

In another paper, the same group demonstrates the applicability of the SWE technique for differentiation between papillary thyroid cancer (PTC) and ET in children [17]. The group studied consisted of 31 subjects, in whom 53 foci of ETs were depicted. The authors expressed the elasticity with a quantitative method. The results demonstrated that the elasticity of ETs is similar or even higher compared to that of the thyroid gland, while SWE proved to be a valuable technique for diagnostics of ET cases. The authors concluded that SWE might allow us to avoid the biopsy at least in some cases, which at the same time should undergo a careful follow-up involving conventional ultrasound examination coupled with SWE assessment.

In the prospective study by Szczepanek-Parulska et al., the potential to differentiate the character of thyroid lesions of new proposed ultrasound-based methods is validated—EU-TIRADS classification and commercially available software S-Detect, and a combinations of both [1]. In the study, 88 patients were included who had been diagnosed with 133 focal lesions, and who were later on subjected to thyroidectomy and/or FNAB. Only those patients in whom unambiguous results of histopathological or cytological examination were obtained were qualified for analysis. S-detect software turned out to be a highly sensitive method, presenting good specificity. The classification of nodules with the use of EU-TIRADS scale turned out to be highly sensitive, though not very specific. The best results in terms of diagnostic performance of malignant lesions were obtained for the S-Detect (when it provided estimation of the "possibly malignant" nodule), while, simultaneously, the lesion gained four or five points or exactly five points in EU-TIRADS scale.

The study by Wieczorek-Szukala et al. encompassed 61 patients diagnosed with PTC, who also underwent $BRAF^{V600E}$ mutation status evaluation [18]. Their results demonstrated that the Snail-1expression correlated with the metastatic potential of PTC. Such an observation was not confirmed with regard to TGFβ1. It was evidenced for the first time that upregulation of Snail-1 corresponded to the presence of $BRAF^{V600E}$ mutation. In addition, authors provided evidence that overexpression of Snail-1 is dependent on $BRAF^{V600E}$ mutation status. In another study, Jensen et al., with the use of microfluidic digital PCR and co-amplification at lower denaturation temperature (COLD) PCR, evaluated the cell-free DNA with *BRAFV600E* mutations (cf*BRAFV600E*) obtained from peripheral blood. The 57 samples from patients diagnosed with PTC harboring somatic *BRAFV600E* mutation were studied [19]. The cf DNA with *BRAFV600E* mutation was found in 42.1% of the studied subjects, while its detection has been demonstrated to correlate with the size of the primary tumor, multifocal form, extrathyroidal spread of the disease and lack of excellent response to treatment if compared to patients with undetectable mutated cf DNA. The studied method has been recently successfully introduced for the evaluation of patients with neoplasms. The authors conclude that the tested method is useful to identify patients presenting higher probability of non-excellet response to therapy, either biochemical or structural, might not be excellent.

The study by Castellnou et al. analyzed the influence of the presurgical management on appropriate evaluation of indications for surgery [20]. The source of data was a nationwide cohort study on patients operated on between 2012 and 2015. Three pathways were distinguished: (1) "FNAB—containing only FNAB, (2) "FNAB+ENDO"—including a consultation by an endocrinologist, (3) "NO FNAB"—FNAB was not performed. Among the 1080 patients, 18.2% underwent "FNAB+ENDO", 19.2%—"FNAB", while 62.6% "NO FNAB". Comparing to "NO FNAB", "FNAB+ENDO" care pathway more frequently was associated with a diagnosis of thyroid cancer (OR 2.67, 1.88–3.81), which was similar to "FNAB" path (OR 2.09, 1.46–2.98). Following thyroidectomies, which were performed at university hospitals, a thyroid cancer diagnosis was established more often (OR 1.61, 1.19–2.17). The recommended care pathway was found to provide more relevant estimation of indications for surgery. The authors noted that although guidelines regarding pre-surgical procedures had not been satisfactorily put into practice, the adherence to recommendations had improved throughout the years.

In another paper, the advantages of the application of intraoperative neuromonitoring of the recurrent laryngeal nerve (IONM) were shown, which, according to authors' findings, reduces the rate of one of the most important complications of thyroid surgeries in bilateral planned thyroidectomies —bilateral vocal cord dysfunction (bVCD) [21]. This retrospective analysis involved prospectively documented data from 20-year experience of a tertiary referral center. Out of 22,573 patients involved in the analysis, only 65 developed bVCD (0.288%). The rate of bVCD was 0.44 prior to the introduction of the routine use of the procedure, and dropped to 0.09% after routine implementation of IONM ($p < 0.001$). In conclusion, taking into consideration the presented results, the authors state that IONM should be recommended for planned and bilateral thyroidectomies. Non-complete bilateral surgery rate after intraoperative non-transient loss of signal in the studied group reached 2%.

In the paper by Smaxwill et al., the potential to identify parathyroid adenomas (PAs) of [^{18}F]fluoro-ethylcholine-PET-CT&4D-CT (FEC-PET&4D-CT) was retrospectively analysed in subjects, in whom ultrasound or MIBI-scintiscan failed to provide direct localisation. In 171 FEC-PET&4D-CTs, the presence of PAs was suggested in 159 of examinations (92.9%). Among 147 patients who already had parathyroidectomy, FEC-PET&4D-CT precisely identified PA in 141 (false negative results in four patients, false positive in two patients). The sensitivity reached 97% and the accuracy reached 96%, while the positive predictive value (PPV) was equal to 99%. Thus, authors conclude that FEC-PET&4D-CT shows exceptional correctness in localization of PAs, where traditional methods are not able to provide accurate localisation [22].

The study by Hung et al. evaluated the role of ultrasound-guided parathormone (PTH) concentration assessment in neck lesions suspected of being PAs in a group of subjects with complicated recurrent or persistent secondary hyperparathyroidism [23]. The authors proposed a new definition for a positive result—PTH washout concentration higher than one-thirtieth of the serum PTH. In the study, 32 patients were included, in whom 50 PTH aspirate concentrations were measured. One-third of 39 washout-positive lesions were not visible on scintigraphic examination. A total of 28 lesions (71.8%) had equivocal ultrasonography results. When the results of histopathological examination following surgical treatment were treated as reference, the PTH aspirate concentration measurement characterized with a 100% PPV. Therefore, the authors suggested that PTH concentration tissue aspirate assessment with the proposed new definition of a positive assay could be very useful to localize PAs in subjects suffering from complicated recurrent or persistent hyperparathyroidism of renal origin.

Interesting findings were also presented by Gawrychowski et al. in a study concerning surgical management of PHP [24]. This was a retrospective clinicopathologic analysis on 1019 patients from a single institution treated throughout a period of 35 years. Treatment failure was observed in 19 cases (1.9%); however, the repeated surgical intervention allowed for achieving remission of the disease in 16 cases. The authors conclude that the ectopic mediastinal location of the PA increases the risk of surgical treatment failure. However, the authors also underline that a majority of PAs of mediastinal localization can still be managed from cervical access.

In conclusion, sonoelastography proves to be a useful method in non-invasive differentiation of thyroid focal lesions in children and adult populations. Simultaneous application of both evaluation of thyroid lesions using EU-TIRADS scale and software based on artificial intelligence yielded the best diagnostic performance in malignancy risk prediction. In terms of progress in evaluation of molecular markers of thyroid cancer, the expression of Snail-1 correlates with the metastatic potential of PTC. Determination of the presence of cell-free DNA harboring *BRAFV600E* mutation in samples obtained from the plasma of patients with PTC using microfluidic digital PCR and COLD PCR provides important information for the prediction of response to therapy and metastatic potential of PTC. If surgical therapy is concerned, an appropriate pathway of selection of patients including FNAB and endocrinologist consultation is necessary to adequately qualify eligible subjects for thyroidectomy. Application of IONM of the recurrent laryngeal nerve may help to decrease the incidence of bilateral vocal cord dysfunction in subjects undergoing planned bilateral thyroidectomies. The progress of localization diagnostics of PAs is achieved by application of [^{18}F]fluoro-ethylcholine-PET-CT&4D-CT and PTH concentration assessment in washout from ultrasound-guided biopsy, which allows for precise localisation of PAs in patients, in whom conventional methods (ultrasonography, MIBI-scintiscan) failed to provide unequivocal results. Surgical experience shows that the parathyroidectomy is successful method of therapy in the vast majority of patients. Although ectopic mediastinal location of PAs may increase the risk of treatment failure, the majority of PAs of mediastinal localization still can be successfully managed from the cervical access.

Author Contributions: Conceptualization, E.S.-P. and M.R.; methodology, E.S.-P. and M.R.; software, E.S.-P. and M.R.; validation, M.R.; formal analysis, M.R.; investigation, E.S.-P.; resources, M.R.; data curation, E.S.-P.; writing—original draft preparation, E.S.-P.; writing—review and editing, M.R.; visualization, E.S.-P.; supervision, M.R.; project administration, M.R. All authors have read and agreed to the published version of the manuscript.

Funding: This research received no external funding.

Conflicts of Interest: The authors declare no conflict of interest.

References

1. Szczepanek-Parulska, E.; Wolinski, K.; Dobruch-Sobczak, K.; Antosik, P.; Ostalowska, A.; Krauze, A.; Migda, B.; Zylka, A.; Lange-Ratajczak, M.; Banasiewicz, T.; et al. S-Detect Software vs. EU-TIRADS Classification: A Dual-Center Validation of Diagnostic Performance in Differentiation of Thyroid Nodules. *J. Clin. Med.* **2020**, *9*, 2495. [CrossRef] [PubMed]
2. Dobruch-Sobczak, K.; Adamczewski, Z.; Szczepanek-Parulska, E.; Migda, B.; Wolinski, K.; Krauze, A.; Prostko, P.; Ruchala, M.; Lewinski, A.; Jakubowski, W.; et al. Histopathological Verification of the Diagnostic Performance of the EU-TIRADS Classification of Thyroid Nodules-Results of a Multicenter Study Performed in a Previously Iodine-Deficient Region. *J. Clin. Med.* **2019**, *8*, 1781. [CrossRef] [PubMed]
3. Kezlarian, B.; Lin, O. Artificial Intelligence in Thyroid Fine Needle Aspiration Biopsies. *Acta Cytol.* **2021**, *65*, 324–329. [CrossRef] [PubMed]
4. Thomas, J.; Haertling, T. AIBx, Artificial Intelligence Model to Risk Stratify Thyroid Nodules. *Thyroid* **2020**, *30*, 878–884. [CrossRef]
5. Zhao, H.B.; Liu, C.; Ye, J.; Chang, L.F.; Xu, Q.; Shi, B.W.; Liu, L.L.; Yin, Y.L.; Shi, B.B. A comparison between deep learning convolutional neural networks and radiologists in the differentiation of benign and malignant thyroid nodules on CT images. *Endokrynol. Pol.* **2021**, *72*, 217–225. [CrossRef]
6. Borowczyk, M.; Szczepanek-Parulska, E.; Olejarz, M.; Wieckowska, B.; Verburg, F.A.; Debicki, S.; Budny, B.; Janicka-Jedynska, M.; Ziemnicka, K.; Ruchala, M. Evaluation of 167 Gene Expression Classifier (GEC) and ThyroSeq v2 Diagnostic Accuracy in the Preoperative Assessment of Indeterminate Thyroid Nodules: Bivariate/HROC Meta-analysis. *Endocr. Pathol.* **2019**, *30*, 8–15. [CrossRef]
7. Wolinski, K.; Stangierski, A.; Szczepanek-Parulska, E.; Gurgul, E.; Budny, B.; Wrotkowska, E.; Biczysko, M.; Ruchala, M. VEGF-C Is a Thyroid Marker of Malignancy Superior to VEGF-A in the Differential Diagnostics of Thyroid Lesions. *PLoS ONE* **2016**, *11*, e0150124. [CrossRef]
8. Mulita, F.; Plachouri, M.K.; Liolis, E.; Vailas, M.; Panagopoulos, K.; Maroulis, I. Patient outcomes following surgical management of thyroid nodules classified as Bethesda category III (AUS/FLUS). *Endokrynol. Pol.* **2021**, *72*, 143–144. [CrossRef]

9. Erturk, M.S.; Cekic, B.; Celik, M.; Demiray Uguz, I. Microwave ablation of autonomously functioning thyroid nodules: A comparative study with radioactive iodine therapy on the functional treatment success. *Endokrynol. Pol.* **2021**, *72*, 120–125. [CrossRef]
10. Kowalski, G.J.; Bula, G.; Zadlo, D.; Gawrychowska, A.; Gawrychowski, J. Primary hyperparathyroidism. *Endokrynol. Pol.* **2020**, *71*, 260–270. [CrossRef]
11. Cyranska-Chyrek, E.; Szczepanek-Parulska, E.; Markuszewski, J.; Kruczynski, J.; Ruchala, M. Sudden Hip Pain in a Young Woman. *Am. J. Med.* **2017**, *130*, e379–e381. [CrossRef] [PubMed]
12. Brominska, B.; Milewska, E.; Szczepanek-Parulska, E.; Czepczynski, R.; Ruchala, M. Diagnostic workup of a patient with severe hypercalcemia and a history of malignancy. *Pol. Arch. Intern. Med.* **2021**, *131*, 727–729. [CrossRef] [PubMed]
13. Silva, B.C.; Cusano, N.E.; Bilezikian, J.P. Primary hyperparathyroidism. *Best Pract. Res. Clin. Endocrinol. Metab.* **2018**, *32*, 593–607. [CrossRef] [PubMed]
14. Gut, P.; Komarowska, H.; Czarnywojtek, A.; Waligorska-Stachura, J.; Baczyk, M.; Ziemnicka, K.; Fischbach, J.; Wrotkowska, E.; Ruchala, M. Familial syndromes associated with neuroendocrine tumours. *Contemp. Oncol.* **2015**, *19*, 176–183. [CrossRef] [PubMed]
15. Press, D.M.; Siperstein, A.E.; Berber, E.; Shin, J.J.; Metzger, R.; Monteiro, R.; Mino, J.; Swagel, W.; Mitchell, J.C. The prevalence of undiagnosed and unrecognized primary hyperparathyroidism: A population-based analysis from the electronic medical record. *Surgery* **2013**, *154*, 1232–1237; discussion 1237–1238. [CrossRef] [PubMed]
16. Adamczewski, Z.; Stasiak, M.; Stasiak, B.; Adamczewska, M.; Lewinski, A. Interobserver Agreement and Plane-Dependent Intraobserver Variability of Shear Wave Sonoelastography in the Differential Diagnosis of Ectopic Thymus Tissue. *J. Clin. Med.* **2021**, *10*, 214. [CrossRef]
17. Stasiak, M.; Adamczewski, Z.; Stawerska, R.; Stasiak, B.; Lewinski, A. Application of Shear Wave Sonoelastography in the Differential Diagnosis of Extra- and Intra-Thyroidal Ectopic Thymic Tissue. *J. Clin. Med.* **2020**, *9*, 3816. [CrossRef]
18. Wieczorek-Szukala, K.; Kopczynski, J.; Kowalska, A.; Lewinski, A. Snail-1 Overexpression Correlates with Metastatic Phenotype in BRAF(V600E) Positive Papillary Thyroid Carcinoma. *J. Clin. Med.* **2020**, *9*, 2701. [CrossRef]
19. Jensen, K.; Thakur, S.; Patel, A.; Mendonca-Torres, M.C.; Costello, J.; Gomes-Lima, C.J.; Walter, M.; Wartofsky, L.; Burman, K.D.; Bikas, A.; et al. Detection of BRAFV600E in Liquid Biopsy from Patients with Papillary Thyroid Cancer Is Associated with Tumor Aggressiveness and Response to Therapy. *J. Clin. Med.* **2020**, *9*, 2481. [CrossRef]
20. Castellnou, S.; Lifante, J.C.; Polazzi, S.; Pascal, L.; Borson-Chazot, F.; Duclos, A. Influence of Care Pathway on Thyroid Nodule Surgery Relevance: A Historical Cohort Study. *J. Clin. Med.* **2020**, *9*, 2271. [CrossRef]
21. Smaxwil, C.; Aleker, M.; Altmeier, J.; Naddaf, A.; Busch, M.; Wagner, J.; Harsch, S.; Ploner, O.; Zielke, A. Neuromonitoring of the Recurrent Laryngeal Nerve Reduces the Rate of Bilateral Vocal Cord Dysfunction in Planned Bilateral Thyroid Procedures. *J. Clin. Med.* **2021**, *10*, 740. [CrossRef] [PubMed]
22. Smaxwil, C.; Aschoff, P.; Reischl, G.; Busch, M.; Wagner, J.; Altmeier, J.; Ploner, O.; Zielke, A. [(18)F]fluoro-ethylcholine-PET Plus 4D-CT (FEC-PET-CT): A Break-Through Tool to Localize the "Negative" Parathyroid Adenoma. One Year Follow Up Results Involving 170 Patients. *J. Clin. Med.* **2021**, *10*, 1648. [CrossRef]
23. Hung, C.L.; Hsu, Y.C.; Huang, S.M.; Hung, C.J. Application of Tissue Aspirate Parathyroid Hormone Assay for Imaging Suspicious Neck Lesions in Patients with Complicated Recurrent or Persistent Renal Hyperparathyroidism. *J. Clin. Med.* **2021**, *10*, 329. [CrossRef] [PubMed]
24. Gawrychowski, J.; Kowalski, G.J.; Bula, G.; Bednarczyk, A.; Zadlo, D.; Niedzielski, Z.; Gawrychowska, A.; Koziolek, H. Surgical Management of Primary Hyperparathyroidism-Clinicopathologic Study of 1019 Cases from a Single Institution. *J. Clin. Med.* **2020**, *9*, 3540. [CrossRef] [PubMed]

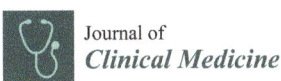

Article

How Long Does It Take to Regain Normocalcaemia in the Event of Postsurgical Hypoparathyroidism? A Detailed Time Course Analysis

Laura Guglielmetti [1,†], Sina Schmidt [1,†], Mirjam Busch [2], Joachim Wagner [2], Ali Naddaf [2], Barbara Leitner [3], Simone Harsch [3], Andreas Zielke [2] and Constantin Smaxwil [2,*]

[1] Department of Surgery, Kantonsspital Winterthur, 8400 Winterthur, Switzerland; laura.guglielmetti@ksw.ch (L.G.); sina.schmidt@ksw.ch (S.S.)
[2] Department of Endocrine Surgery, Endocrine Center Stuttgart, Diakonie-Klinikum Stuttgart, 70176 Stuttgart, Germany; buschm@diak-stuttgart.de (M.B.); wagner@diak-stuttgart.de (J.W.); naddaf@diak-stuttgart.de (A.N.); andreas.zielke@diak-stuttgart.de (A.Z.)
[3] Outcomes Research Unit, Endocrine Center Stuttgart, Diakonie-Klinikum Stuttgart, 70176 Stuttgard, Germany; leitner-barbara@t-online.de (B.L.); simone.harsch@diak-stuttgart.de (S.H.)
* Correspondence: smaxwil@diak-stuttgart.de
† These authors contributed equally to this work.

Abstract: Background: Postsurgical hypoparathyroidism (PH) is the most common side effect of bilateral thyroid resections. Data regarding the time course of recovery from PH are currently unavailable. Therefore, a detailed analysis of the time course of PH recovery and conditions associated with rapid recovery was conducted. Methods: This is a retrospective analysis of prospectively documented data. Patients with biochemical signs of PH or need for calcium supplementation were followed-up for 12 months. Logistic regression analyses were used to identify covariates of early as opposed to late recovery from PH. Results: There were 1097 thyroid resections performed from 06/2015 to 07/2016 with n = 143 PH. Median recovery time was 8 weeks and six patients (1.1% of total thyroid resections) required calcium supplementation > 12 months. Recovery of PH within 4 and 12 weeks was characterized by high PTH levels on the first postoperative day (4 weeks: OR 1.13, 95% CI 1.06–1.20; 12 weeks: OR 1.08, 95%CI 1.01–1.16). Visualization of all PTGs emerged as an independent predictor of recovery within 12 months (OR 2.32, 95% CI 1.01–4.93) and 24 weeks (OR 2.69, 95% CI 1.08–6.69). Conclusion: In the setting of specialized high-volume endocrine surgery, permanent PH is rare. However, every second patient will require more than 2 months of continued medical surveillance. Early recovery was associated with only moderately decreased postsurgical PTH-levels. Successful late recovery appeared to be associated with the number of parathyroid glands visualized during surgery.

Keywords: thyroid surgery; postsurgical hypoparathyroidism; risk-factor analysis; time course

1. Introduction

Postsurgical hypoparathyroidism (PH) is the most common complication following total thyroidectomy [1]. PH impairs a patient's convalescence and prolongs outpatient follow-up [2,3]. Patients experiencing PH require increased medical attention, repeated biochemical assessment, as well as additional medication, all of which affect medical resource use. Moreover, patients with severe, persisting PH often suffer incapacitating symptoms and are likely to be confronted with a reduced quality of life, as well as reduced life expectancy [4].

At present, no consensus exists for the definition of PH, nor for the interval until PH might have to be considered a permanent condition. Traditional cut-offs for permanent PH are either 6 [5–12] or 12 months [1,2,13]. Most authors use biochemical definitions for PH, such as PTH levels (with different cut-offs) [1] or postoperative hypocalcemia [12–15]. Less

Citation: Guglielmetti, L.; Schmidt, S.; Busch, M.; Wagner, J.; Naddaf, A.; Leitner, B.; Harsch, S.; Zielke, A.; Smaxwil, C. How Long Does It Take to Regain Normocalcaemia in the Event of Postsurgical Hypoparathyroidism? A Detailed Time Course Analysis. *J. Clin. Med.* **2022**, *11*, 3202. https://doi.org/10.3390/jcm11113202

Academic Editor: Neveen Agnes Therese Hamdy

Received: 29 March 2022
Accepted: 1 June 2022
Published: 3 June 2022

Publisher's Note: MDPI stays neutral with regard to jurisdictional claims in published maps and institutional affiliations.

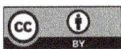

Copyright: © 2022 by the authors. Licensee MDPI, Basel, Switzerland. This article is an open access article distributed under the terms and conditions of the Creative Commons Attribution (CC BY) license (https://creativecommons.org/licenses/by/4.0/).

frequently, newly prescribed postoperative calcium and/or vitamin D supplementation are taken as a surrogate to characterize the event of PH as a hormonal insufficiency state.

However, data regarding the course of convalescence after PH are scarce, and to the best of our knowledge, a detailed analysis of individual time courses of recovery from PH, as well as the clinical and biochemical data associated with the length of the period of convalescence are currently not available. Such insight would be highly desirable to allow for the optimum allocation of resources. Determining the expected time course of individual PH recovery could facilitate identifying patients who are dependent on prolonged and experienced medical support and, therefore, may benefit from specialized medical professionals.

Therefore, this study conducted a detailed analysis of the biochemical recovery of patients with PH. Moreover, this study aimed to identify predictors for early recovery (i.e., 4 weeks), as well as for prolonged (i.e., more than 24 and 52 weeks) postoperative hypocalcemia.

2. Materials and Methods

2.1. Study Population

We performed a selective analysis of prospectively documented data of a consecutive series of patients undergoing thyroid surgeries at a specialized centre of Endocrine Surgery. Datasets of the registry, medical charts, as well as data from the Centres' structured follow-up program were analysed including all patients undergoing thyroid surgeries in this institution between June 2015 and May 2016. With regard to the datasets until discharge of an individual patient, there were no missing values. Patients with co-existing parathyroid pathology diagnosed either preoperatively or incidentally during surgery for a thyroid pathology were excluded from this analysis (n = 64 of which n = 23 total thyroidectomy, n = 26 hemithyroidectomies, and n = 15 other procedures).

All individuals in this series underwent surgery at a high-volume centre of reference in thyroid and parathyroid surgery, certified by the German Association of Surgery (DGAV) [16]. All operations were attended by a certified Endocrine Surgeon, using highly standardized surgical protocols with a focus to apply minimal invasive techniques whenever possible. These techniques do not mandate extensive dissection to visualize all four parathyroid glands, but encourage the demonstration and preservation of at least one parathyroid gland during the procedure. Moreover, parathyroid glands that were attached to the thyroid lobe and could not be preserved in situ were routinely dissected and subject to auto-transplantation into the ipsilateral sternocleidoid muscle. In accordance with current practice guidelines, conventional medical therapy of PH always involved the concomitant use of calcium supplements and active vitamin D preparation (i.e., Calcitriol; 1.25 (OH)2D3; 0.25–0.5 µg bid).

2.2. Postsurgical Follow-up Data

All patients in this series were subject to a standardized perioperative recovery protocol, ensuring biochemical testing for fasting (total serum) calcium, and PTH levels between 7 and 8 a.m. on post-operative day (POD) 1 and POD2, as well as POD3 in the rare event a patient had not yet been discharged. Calcium and PTH levels were determined using a Cobas pro (Cobas e 801) from Roche (ECLIA, intact PTH: normal range 15 to 65 pg/mL; total serum calcium normal range 2.2–2.6 mmol/L).

All patients with either symptoms of PH or biochemically proven hypocalcaemia and/or hypoprothrombinaemia or newly prescribed calcium plus vitamin D (i.e., 1,25 (OH)2D3) medication were defined as potential candidates for PH and subjected to a detailed follow-up program. To this end, the Endocrine Centers Outcomes Research Unit used regular (i.e., monthly) structured telephone interviews to assess current medication (specifically: calcium supplements and vitamin D3), laboratory parameters, and symptoms of hypocalcemia. Follow-up was terminated only if a full recovery had been validated by the biochemical demonstration of normocalcaemia, as well as euparathormonaemia (as determined by the respective local assay or test) and the individual was without oral calcium intake. For the purpose of this paper, 12-month results were analysed. In the event a patient was "lost to follow-up" after multiple unsuccessful calls, the last observation was carried on forward and the outcome documented accordingly (LOCF).

2.3. Definition of Postsurgical Hypoparathyroidism

Historically, the duration of PH is termed and classified taking account of two different intervals: transient PH, i.e., PH lasting for less than 12 or less than 24 weeks, and permanent PH for cases lasting longer than either 6 or 12 months. This is also found in most clinical guidelines [1,5–10,13,17,18]. Hence, predictors of the duration of PH were determined using logistic regression analysis at these specific time points: 12, 24, and more than 24 weeks after surgery. In accordance with current guidelines, all cases with clinical signs of hypocalcaemia or need for calcium and active vitamin D (i.e., Calcitirol; 1,25 (OH)2D3) medication or biochemically proven hypocalcaemia and/or hypoprothrombinaemia persisting for more than twelve months after surgery were defined to have "permanent hypoparathyroidism" [1,5–10,13,17,18].

2.4. Handling of Data and Statistical Analysis

All perioperative data were prospectively documented as individual datasets according to the thyroid-surgery-module of the StuDoQ-Quality Assurance Registry of the German Surgical Association (DGAV) after informed consent [16]. All data computed for this publication were pseudonymized or aggregate non-individual data. Descriptive statistics was used to summarize patients' characteristics. Continuous variables are reported as the mean and standard deviation (SD) or median and interquartile range and were compared between groups using two-sample independent t-tests or Mann–Whitney U-tests (non-normal data). Categorical variables were summarized as frequencies (%) and compared using Pearson's chi-squared test or Fisher's exact test where applicable.

The variables included for univariate analysis in the logistic regression models were a priori determined after literature review. A total of n = 8 variables were tested in univariable models: gender, presence of Graves' disease, malignant thyroid conditions, visualization of all parathyroid glands during thyroid surgery, reimplantation of parathyroid glands, PTH and calcium on POD 1, and symptoms of hypocalcemia. Variables with a *p*-value of <0.15 were retained in the multivariable models. All variables retained in the multivariable models had no more than a weak correlation (Spearman correlation coefficient r < 0.39, as suggested by Evans et al.) [19]. In this cohort of patients, there was no strong correlation between female gender and presence of graves' disease (Spearman correlation coefficient r = 0.147, *p* = 0.079).

Results are reported as the odds ratio (OR) with the corresponding 95% confidence interval (CI). Goodness of fit was tested using the Hosmer–Lemeshow test, and the area under the curve (AUC) is reported for the predictive accuracy of the model. SPSS version 25 (IBM corp., Armonk, NY, USA) and R Studio Version 3.2.1. (RStudio, Inc., Boston, MA, USA) were used for data analysis. *p*-values < 0.05 (two-tailed) were considered statistically significant.

2.5. Ethics Approval and Consent to Participate

This study was approved by the Institutional Review Board of the Diakonie-Klinikum Stuttgart and conducted in cooperation with the Endocrine Centers certified Outcomes Research Unit. All methods were carried out in accordance with the Declaration of Helsinki and the approved guidelines. As mentioned, data enrolled in this study were obtained from the StuDoQ quality assurance database, for which informed consent had been obtained. The data presented in this article do not represent a human participant research study and do not include personal identifying information. This secondary analysis was carried out for the purpose of quality assurance and did not require informed consent.

3. Results

During the 12-month period, a total of 1097 + 69 surgeries for thyroid pathologies were performed. There were 69 cases that had to be excluded because of co-existing parathyroid pathologies with removal of at least one parathyroid gland. Thyroid resections comprised 538 complete resections (505 total thyroidectomies (TTX) and 33 two-staged thyroidectomies) and 559 less-than-total resections (515 hemithyroidectomies and 44 comprising of central resections, as well as bilateral subtotal resections such as Hartley, Dunhill, Enderlein–Hotz). The patient characteristics of all procedures are displayed in Table 1. Of all thyroid patients, 74.5% were female, and 85.9% had benign conditions including 86 patients with Graves' disease, all of which had total thyroidectomies (7.8% of the entire cohort, 15.9% of TTX). A total of n = 155 patients had malignant thyroid pathologies (14.1% of the entire cohort, 27.9% of TTX), of which 67 patients had a systematic dissection of cervical lymph nodes involving Robbins-Regions VI and VII (6.1% of the cohort, 12.8% of TTX). There were 126 patients with previous surgery to the neck (rate of reoperations: 11.5%). Surgery for recurrent benign goitre was recorded in 54 cases (4.9%). Of these, nine had bilateral and the remainder unilateral reoperations (83.3%).

Table 1. Baseline characteristics for all patients and all patients with postsurgical hypoparathyroidism.

n (%) Unless Otherwise Stated	All Procedures n = 1097	Procedures w Postsurgical Hypoparathyroidism (PH) n = 143
Malignant thyroid condition	155 (14.1)	20 (14)
Central LAD	67 (6.1)	22 (16.8)
Graves' disease	86 (7.8)	16 (11.2)
Reoperative Surgery	126 (11.5)	12 (8.4)
Thyroidectomy	505 (46)	127 (88.8)
Hemithyroidectomy (HTx)	515 (46.9)	2 (1.4)
Two-staged bilateral HTx	33 (3.0)	14 (9.8)
PTG visualised		
0	71 (6.5)	7 (4.9)
1	205 (18.7)	3 (3.1)
2	390 (35.6)	22 (15.4)
3	152 (13.9)	43 (30.1)
4	279 (25.4)	68 (47.5)
PTG autograft		
0	938 (85.5)	110 (76.9)
1	146 (13.3)	31 (21.7)
2	12 (1.1)	2 (1.4)
4	1 (0.1)	0
PTH POD 1, median (IQR)	-	10.4 (8.1–14.4)
PTH POD 2, median (IQR)	-	9.8 (7.6–11.9)
Calcium POD 1, median (IQR)	-	2.1 (2.0–2.2)
Calcium POD 2, median (IQR)	-	2.0 (1.9–2.1)

Abbreviations: LAD = lymphadenectomy, POD = postoperative day, PTG = parathyroid glands, PTH = parathyroid hormone; IQR = interquartile range.

There were 154 patients with either newly prescribed calcium and vitamin D (i.e., Calcitriol; 1,25 $(OH)_2D_3$) medication or hypocalcaemia or hypoprothrombinaemia or hypocalcaemic symptoms on any postoperative day. Of these, 11 had to be excluded because of incomplete data (n = 2) or because they were not willing to be entered into the follow-up program (n = 9), leaving 143 patients for analysis (92%).

3.1. Postsurgical Hypocalcaemia—Patient Characteristics

The majority of patients with PH were female n = 122 (88.3%); n = 127 (88.8%) had undergone total thyroidectomy (see Table 1 and Figure 1), and n = 14 (9.8%) patients had a two-stage thyroidectomy. One patient (0.7%) had unilateral hemithyroidectomy plus subtotal resection of the contralateral lobe, while another patient (0.7%) had a unilateral hemithyroidectomy and no history of thyroid surgery in the past. Both of them had lowered PTH levels and symptoms of hypocalcaemia on POD1.

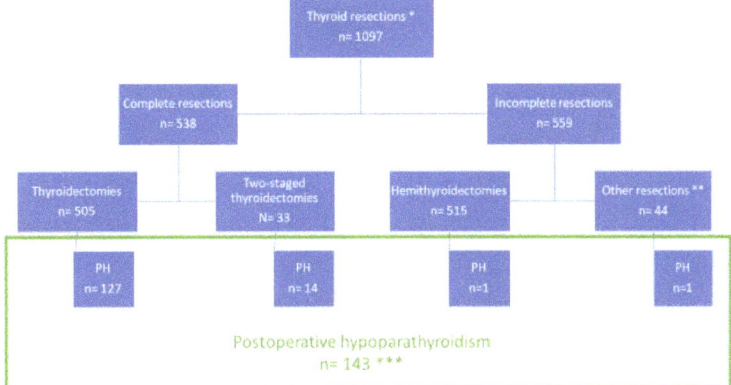

Figure 1. Overview of the extent of resection in patients included into the study. * There were that 69 had to be excluded due to co-existing parathyroid pathologies with removal of at least one parathyroid gland, leaving 1097 for analysis; ** comprising central resections, as well as bilateral subtotal resections such as Hartley, Dunhill, Enderlein–Hotz; *** patients with complete datasets.

Histopathological diagnoses confirmed benign thyroid conditions in 123 and included 16 patients with Graves' disease (11.2%) and 12 redo-operations (8.4%). There were 20 patients confirmed to have thyroid cancer (14%), and a dissection of the central cervical lymph nodes had been carried out in 22 patients (16.8%).

Parathyroid gland visualization was recorded in all of the cases, with one gland documented in three (3.1%), two glands in 22 (15.4%), three glands in 43 (30.1%), and four glands in 68 patients (47.5%), respectively. There were seven patients in whom no parathyroid gland had been visualized (4.9%). Parathyroid gland auto-transplantation was recorded in n = 33 (23.1%) patients and involved one gland in n = 31 (94%) and two glands in n = 2 (6%). These data were not different from the entire cohort of bilateral procedures (Table 1).

Of 143 patients, 81 (56.6%) reported symptoms of hypocalcaemia on any given day during the postoperative course (Figure 2). Likewise, 63 (44.1%) had calcium of less than 2.0 mmol/l (normal range 2.0–2.75 mmol/l), of which n = 23 had calcium of less than 2.0 mmol/l on POD 1. Of all patients, 114 (79.7%) had a PTH level below the lower limit of norm (iPTH-assay range 15–65 pg/mL), and of these, 109 had a PTH of <15 pg/mL recorded on POD 1. Calcium glucoronate starting at the same day of the surgical procedure had been ordered in 15 cases (10.5%). Of these cases, n = 2 had undergone hemithyroidectomy because of recurrent benign nodular goitre, n = 3 had a total thyroidectomy with central lymph node clearance for thyroid cancer, n = 2 had a total thyroidectomy for Graves' disease, and n = 4 had at least one autografted parathyroid gland. Symptoms of hypocalcemia, albeit with a normal biochemical parameter, had been recorded in n = 6. However, taking account of the entire period of postoperative hospitalization, all but two patients (n = 141) had been ordered postoperative calcium supplementation until discharge. Two patients chose not to take supplementary calcium medication despite symptoms of hypocalcaemia.

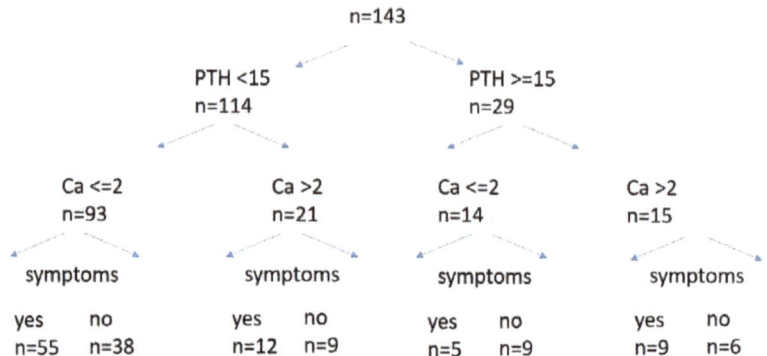

Figure 2. Overview of biochemical and clinical findings in patients with postsurgical hypoparathyroidism. Roche Cobas pro e 801; intact PTH = parathyroid hormone (ECLIA; 15 to 65 pg/mL), Ca = total serum calcium (2.2–2.6 mmol/L).

3.2. Postsurgical Hypoparathyroidism—Time Course of Recovery

Median recovery time of PH for all patients was 8 weeks, and two thirds of all patients recovered within 18 weeks (IQR 4–18 weeks). As depicted in Figure 2, the slope of the curve of recovery was steepest and displayed almost linear degression in the first and second 4-week intervals post-surgery. During this period, 50% of patients had a biochemical recovery, whereas the next 25% of patients took more than twice that long for full recovery from PH. Of the 15 patients that had been ordered calcium and vitamin D3 to be initiated immediately after surgery and prior to any biochemical analysis, all had biochemical signs of hypoparathyroidism, and all of them recovered (1 to 33 weeks). Biochemical recovery could not be proven in 3 three patients who were free of symptoms and off calcium and vitamin D, but had self-terminated the follow-up after a median of 16 weeks (IQR 15–17) without any further laboratory testing. Only one patient (0.7% of the cohort, 0.2% of TTX and 0.09% of all thyroid surgeries) required calcium substitution for more than 12 months (Figure 3).

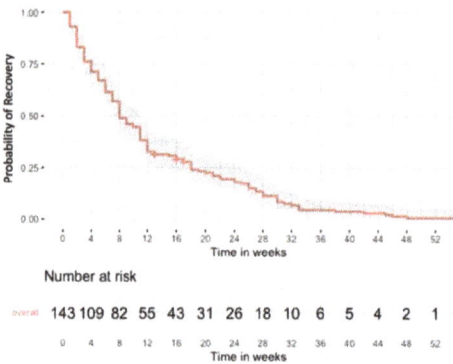

Figure 3. Time to recovery for the entire cohort of patients with postsurgical hypoparathyroidism (Kaplan–Meier).

Historically and currently presented in the respective guidelines, PH is termed transient whenever full recovery occurs either within 12 or within 24 weeks, and it is considered persistent if a biochemical recovery is not documented at 24 weeks [1,5–10,17] or after a period of 12 months [13,18]. In order to interpret potential predictors for the duration or recovery of PH, these intervals were, therefore, taken into account.

Baseline characteristics of patients with a documented recovery within 12 weeks as compared to more than 12 weeks are summarized in Table 2, and those for recovery within 24 weeks as compared to a later recovery are presented in Table 3. Median PTH on POD1 was significantly higher for patients with earlier recovery of PH in each of these groups. Patients with a full recovery within 12 weeks showed a higher PTH level on POD1 than those that took longer (median 11.1 (IQR 7.3–11.6) vs. 9.1 (IQR 9–15.4), p = 0.006). Likewise, PTH levels were higher in those individuals in whom full recovery was documented within 24 weeks as opposed to longer than 24 weeks to recovery (median 10.8 (8.45–15.1) vs. 8.8 (7.3–12.7), p = 0.003). Of note, there was a steady decline of POD1 PTH levels when computed against time to recovery, suggesting that besides predicting the incident, PTH levels (or percentage decline as compared to presurgical levels) may allow for an estimation of individual recovery times (Figure 4).

Table 2. Baseline characteristics for recovery within 12 weeks compared to a later recovery.

n (%) Unless Otherwise Stated	Recovered ≤ 12 Weeks n = 96	Recovered > 12 Weeks n = 47	p-Value
Female gender	85 (88.5)	37 (78.7)	0.136
Thyroidectomy	85 (88.5)	42 (89.4)	1
Graves' disease	14 (14.6)	2 (4.3)	0.09
Malignant thyroid condition	13 (13.5)	7 (14.9)	0.803
Central LND	15 (15.6)	9 (19.1)	0.637
Reoperative surgery	5 (10.6)	7 (7.3)	0.53
PTG visualised			
0	5 (5.2)	2 (4.3)	
1	3 (3.1)	0	
2	11 (11.5)	11 (23.4)	0.066
3	25 (26)	18 (38.3)	
4	52 (54.2)	16 (34)	
PTG autograft			
0	77 (80.2)	33 (70.2)	
1	17 (17.7)	14 (29.8)	0.223
2	2 (2.1)	0	
Immediate calcium substitution	13 (13.5)	2 (4.3)	0.144
Symptoms of PH	55 (57.3)	26 (55.3)	0.859
PTH POD 1, median (IQR)	11.0 (7.3–11.6)	9.1 (9–15.4)	**0.006**
PTH POD 2, median (IQR)	10.2 (7.8–13.6)	8.6 (7.8–12.2)	**0.008**
Calcium POD 1, median (IQR)	2.1 (2–1.1)	2.1 (2–2.2)	0.544
Calcium POD 2, median (IQR)	2 (1.9–2.1)	2 (1.9–2.1)	0.31

Abbreviations: LAD = lymphadenectomy, POD = postoperative day, PTG = parathyroid glands, PTH = parathyroid hormone; IQR = interquartile range.

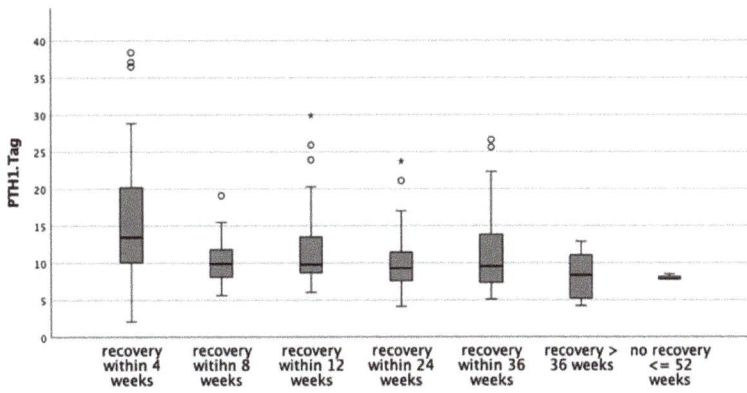

Figure 4. PTH—level on the first postoperative day and time of biochemical recovery from postsurgical hypoparathyroidism. * extreme value, ° outlier.

Table 3. Baseline characteristics for recovery within 24 weeks compared to a later recovery.

n (%) Unless Otherwise Stated	Recovered ≤ 24 Weeks n = 116	Recovered > 24 Weeks n = 27	p-Value
Female gender	98 (84.5)	24 (88.9)	0.765
Thyroidectomy	104 (89.7)	23 (85.2)	0.592
Malignant thyroid condition	16 (13.8)	4 (14.8)	1
Central LAD	17 (14.7)	7 (25.9)	0.163
Graves' disease	15 (12.9)	1 (3.7)	0.307
Reoperative surgery	8 (6.9)	4 (14.8)	0.24
PTG visualised			0.089
0	5 (4.3)	2 (7.4)	0.62
1	3 (2.6)	0	1
2	15 (12.9)	7 (25.9)	0.135
3	33 (28.4)	10 (37.0)	0.485
4	60 (51.7)	8 (29.6)	0.053
PTG autograft			
0	90 (77.6)	20 (74.1)	
1	24 (20.7)	7 (25.9)	1
2	2 (1.7)	0	
Immediate calcium substitution	14 (12.1)	1 (3.7)	0.304
Symptoms of PH	68 (58.6)	13 (48.1)	0.39
PTH POD 1, median (IQR)	10.8 (8.45–15.1)	8.8 (7.3–12.7)	**0.033**
PTH POD 2, median (IQR)	9.9 (7.78–12.53)	8.4 (7–10.45)	0.057
PTH > 15 and <65 POD 1	48 (42.1)	7 (25.9)	0.132
PTH ≥ 10 POD 1	54 (46.6)	18 (66.7)	0.086
Calcium POD 1, median (IQR)	2.1 (2–2.2)	2.0 (2–2.1)	0.096
Calcium POD 2, median (IQR)	2 (1.9–2.1)	1.95 (1.8–2.1)	0.387

Abbreviations: LAD = lymphadenectomy, POD = postoperative day, PTG = parathyroid glands, PTH = parathyroid hormone.

Calcium levels on POD1 or POD2, number of patients with hypocalcaemic symptoms, and percentage of patients undergoing total thyroidectomy per group were not statistically different (Figure 5). This may in part be due to the early and frequent use of perioperative calcium and vitamin D3 substitution in this study.

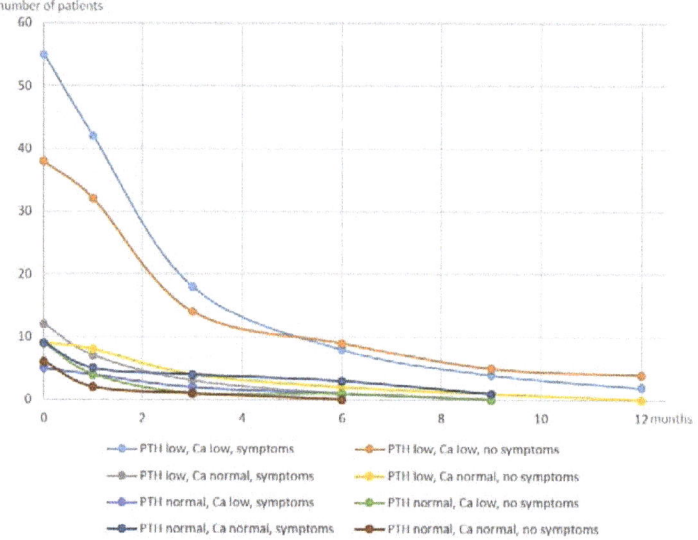

Figure 5. Time to recovery from postsurgical hypoparathyroidism—depicted according to the eight groups shown in Figure 2.

3.3. Postsurgical Hypoparathyroidism—Predictors for Time to Recovery

In order to further explore the utility of clinicopathological variables to predict time to recovery, patients were stratified according to time to recovery and potential predictors of recovery assessed using logistic regression analysis as described above.

The presence of graves' disease, thyroid cancer diagnosis, visualization of the number of parathyroid glands, replantation of parathyroid glands, PTH, and calcium level on POD 1, as well as symptoms of hypocalcemia were tested by univariate analysis and retained in the model in the case of a $p < 0.015$.

A total of n = 41 patients (28.7%) recovered within 4 weeks after surgery. PTH on POD1 emerged as a significant predictor for early recovery (OR 1.13 (95% CI 1.06–1.2) $p < 0.001$) when controlled for Graves' disease and visualization of all PGs (Table 3).

Transient PH, defined as recovery within 12 weeks after surgery, was recorded in n = 96 patients. Visualization of all PGs (OR 2.3 (95% CI 1.01–4.93), $p = 0.029$) and PTH on POD1 (OR 1.08 (95% CI 1.01–1.16), $p = 0.034$) were significant predictors for recovery within three months (Table 4).

Table 4. Logistic regression analysis of potential risk factors.

	Univariable Analysis				Multivariable Analysis			
	OR	Lower CI	Upper CI	p-Value	OR	Lower CI	Upper CI	p-Value
(a) recovery within 4 weeks (within 4 weeks n = 41 vs. later than 4 weeks n = 102)								
Graves' disease	3.82	1.32	11.08	0.014	2.40	0.72	8.07	0.156
Central LAD	0.61	0.21	1.75	0.355				
All PTG visualized	1.86	0.89	3.88	0.097	2.02	0.88	4.63	0.098
PTG autograft	1.35	0.64	2.89	0.433				
PTH POD 1	1.12	1.05	1.19	<0.001	1.13	1.06	1.20	<0.001
Calcium POD 1	0.40	0.03	4.70	0.464				
Symptoms	1.12	0.54	2.32	0.772				
Female gender	2.71	0.75	9.77	0.127	2.69	0.64	11.34	0.178
HL ChiSq 13.966, p 0.083, AUC 0.771								
(b) recovery within 24 weeks (within 12 weeks n = 116 vs. later than 24 weeks n = 27)								
Graves' disease	3.86	0.49	30.3	0.201				
Malignity	0.92	0.28	3.01	0.890				
All PTG visualized	2.55	1.03	6.29	0.043	2.69	1.08	6.69	**0.033**
PTG autograft	0.92	0.38	2.25	0.856				
PTH POD 1	1.07	0.98	1.16	0.136	1.07	0.98	1.16	0.125
Ca POD 1	7.04	0.40	125.0	0.184				
Symptoms	0.65	0.28	1.52	0.325				
Female gender	0.68	0.19	2.50	0.562				
HL ChiSq 7.267, p 0.508, AUC 0.664								

Within 24 weeks following surgery. n = 116 patients had recovered from PH, while the remaining n = 27 patients remained on calcium supplementation for 25–56 weeks, and n = 3 patients were on continued calcium supplementation (i.e., did not recover) after 12-month follow-up. Univariable and multivariable logistic regression analysis revealed visualization of all PGs as a significant predictor of recovery within 24 weeks (OR 2.69 (95% CI 1.08–6.69), $p = 0.033$) when controlled for PTH levels on POD1. While PTH on POD 1 evolved as a predictor of early recovery of PH, later recovery was associated with visualization of all PTGs during surgery when controlled for Graves' disease and female gender.

4. Discussion

Postoperative hypocalcaemia due to impaired parathyroid function is the most common complication after total thyroidectomy. Although much less frequent, permanent hypoparathyroidism imposes an important medical burden—due to the need for additional medication, regular medical visits, and thus, also significant long-term costs [20]. There is still no consensus with regard to the definition of postoperative hypoparathyroidism (PH), nor the time period after which PH may have to be considered a permanent condition.

Much of the uncertainty is due to a lack of data regarding potential causes of PH, risk factors of PH, as well as the time-course and likelihood of reconvalescence from PH. For instance, a recent "raise-your-hand survey" carried out during the British Association of Endocrine and Thyroid Surgeons (BAETS) meeting in Barcelona revealed only some 10% of the attending 220 surgeons to know their rate of inadvertent parathyroidectomy [21].

However, most guidelines use cut-offs for permanent PH of either 6 months [5–12] or 12 months [1,2,13]. Clinical studies use biochemical definitions for PH such as PTH levels, albeit a variety of different cut-offs, or (total) calcium levels, again using a range of cut-off levels. Moreover, by virtue of the variety of PH definitions, the published rate of symptomatic hypocalcaemia varies between 0.1% and 20.2%, and biochemical hypocalcaemia is reported to occur at a rate of 15–75% [12–15,22]. Despite these variations, a recent review found no difference of the incidence of PH at 6 versus 12 months (4.11% and 4.08%) [23].

Some studies have used more inclusive definitions for PH [2,3], arguing that postoperative supplementation of calcium and/or newly started active vitamin D (Calcitriol; 1,25 (OH)2D3) medication affect biochemical and clinical findings. On the basis of this inclusive definition of PH, we found the overall incidence in this consecutive series of patients undergoing bilateral thyroid procedures for a wide array of thyroid pathologies to be 24.5% in bilateral procedures. While almost all of the affected patients had at least one level of total serum calcium below the range of normal (98.6%), symptomatic hypocalcemia was less frequent, occurring in 57% of patients with PH, i.e., 13.7% of bilateral procedures.

Overall, we determined the recovery rate of PH at 6 and 12 months to be 82% and 98%, and there was only one patient who did not fully recover within 12 months (0.7%). Bilezikian et al. reported rates for PH at 24 weeks ranging between 0.9% and 1.6% in centres with a record of excellence in endocrine surgery and suggested the 6-month time period to be sufficient to ascertain permanent postoperative hypoparathyroidism [6]. Others have published rates of permanent PH ranging from 0.5% to 8.6% [1,2,10,11,13] and rates of recovery ranging from 6.9% to 46%, again using a broad range of definitions [6,17]. However, besides such "endpoint-observations" at either 6 or 12 months, the current literature does not offer any insight into the actual time course of recovery from PH.

For the first time, we are now able to report a median recovery time for PH of 8 weeks (IQR 4–18). Almost two thirds of patients with PH had a documented recovery within 12 weeks, and some 8% of all patients with bilateral thyroid procedures required continued medical surveillance for more than 12 weeks. However, some 15% of patients with PH, i.e., 3.5% of all patients with bilateral thyroid procedures, take longer than 6 months to recover.

With regard to prognostic factors of recovery, one of the first prospective studies to suggest postoperative PTH levels, specifically the magnitude of decrease, to be a significant predictor of time to recovery was published by Al Dhahri et al. Their study included n = 53 patients undergoing total thyroidectomy. The authors found 15 (28.5%) of their patients to have PH [1], comparing well to the rate in this current study. A large systematic review of 69 studies did, however, not confirm a particular PTH threshold, neither as a predictor of the prevalence, nor the duration of PH [24]. A recent retrospective study using predefined PTH thresholds suggested the combination of postoperative PTH plus calcium levels to be better predictors of the likelihood of PH [25].

In the present study, median PTH levels on POD1 were significantly higher in patients with earlier recovery, and PTH on POD1 emerged as a significant predictor for early recovery within 4 weeks, as well as for recovery within 12 weeks. Moreover, we determined an increasing probability of an earlier recovery with each increment of PTH on POD1. For patients in whom we had observed longer recovery, e.g., more than 12 weeks, intraoperative visualization of (all) parathyroid glands (PGs) was significantly associated with recovery and remained the only significant predictor of recovery for patients with a recovery period of 24 weeks. Although these observations clearly suggest the intraoperative visualization of PGs to be linked to a late likelihood of recovery, we believe that extensive dissection to demonstrate PGs during surgery is not warranted. Indeed, as had already been emphasized by others, this carries the potential to increase the rate of patients experiencing PH (13,23). It has, however, recently been suggested that taking account of the number of PGs in situ together with measurements calcium and PTH during the first month post thyroidectomy may allow predicting a swift parathyroid recovery [13,21,26,27].

Clearly, one of the limitations of this work is the retrospective character. Because this is a representation of a real-world cohort, data regarding preoperative calcium levels, corrected or ionized calcium values, preoperative medication, or preoperative vitamin D levels were not consistent enough to allow for proper evaluation. This might have been worthwhile, since preoperative vitamin D deficiency has been identified as a possible risk factor of PH [28]. Moreover, as a result of the inclusion criteria of the present study, there is a lack of data from "controls", so no conclusion can be drawn with regard to the association of postoperative PTH levels with the incidence of PH.

However, this is the first report of a detailed time course analysis of recovery from PH in a larger cohort of patients with this condition. Based on the findings, a 6-month cut-off to ascertain permanent PH appears to be inappropriate. However, the majority of patients will recover from PH within 8–12 weeks. The time course detailed in this study should allow for better counselling and planning of out-patient treatment.

Nevertheless, postoperative hypoparathyroidism continues to be a challenge, and it remains to be shown to what extent new techniques such as autofluorescence and fluorescence angiography of the parathyroid glands may lead to an improvement.

5. Conclusions

Permanent hypoparathyroidism is a rare event in the hands of specialized high-volume endocrine surgeons. Transient hypoparathyroidism is, however, observed in every fourth patient with a total thyroidectomy. In every second patient, restoration of normocalcaemia and euparathormonaemia required more than 2 months of continued medical surveillance. Early recovery was more likely if postsurgical PTH levels were only slightly decreased. When recovery took longer, full recovery appeared to be associated with the number of parathyroid glands visualized during surgery.

Author Contributions: Conceptualization, L.G., S.S., A.Z. and C.S.; methodology, L.G., S.S., B.L., A.Z. and C.S.; software, L.G. and A.Z.; validation, L.G., S.S., B.L., A.Z. and C.S.; resources, L.G., S.S., M.B., J.W., A.N. and S.H.; data curation, M.B., A.N., J.W. and S.H.; writing—original draft preparation, L.G., S.S., A.Z. and C.S.; writing—final review and editing, L.G., S.S., M.B., A.Z. and C.S.; visualization, L.G., S.S., J.W. and M.B. All authors have read and agreed to the published version of the manuscript.

Funding: This research received no external funding.

Institutional Review Board Statement: This study was approved by the Institutional Review Board of the Diakonie-Klinikum Stuttgart and conducted by the Endocrine Centers certified Outcomes Research Unit. All methods were carried out in accordance with the Declaration of Helsinki and the approved guidelines. The data enrolled in this study were obtained from the centres pseudonymized quality assurance database (since 2017 the StuDoQ-Database for certified centres of Endocrine Surgery of the German Association of Surgeons, DGAVC).

Informed Consent Statement: Ethical committees determined that the data presented in this article do not represent a human participant research study and do not include personal identifying information and that the study was carried out in accordance with the relevant legislation for the purpose of quality monitoring and quality assurance. Therefore, this analysis did not require informed consent other than the consent obtained prior to entering data into the StuDoQ Database.

Data Availability Statement: Restrictions apply to the data presented in this study. Data were obtained from the StuDoQ Thyroid Quality Assurance Registry of the German Association of Surgeons (DGAVC) and may be available to third parties only upon request to the SAVC/DGAVC and the decision at the discretion of the DGAVC.

Conflicts of Interest: The authors declare no conflict of interest.

References

1. Al-Dhahri, S.F.; Mubasher, M.; Mufarji, K.; Allam, O.S.; Terkawi, A.S. Factors predicting post-thyroidectomy hypoparathyroidism recovery. *World J. Surg.* **2014**, *38*, 2304–2310. [CrossRef] [PubMed]
2. Glinoer, D.; Andry, G.; Chantrain, G.; Samil, N. Clinical aspects of early and late hypocalcaemia afterthyroid surgery. *Eur. J. Surg. Oncol.* **2000**, *26*, 571–577. [CrossRef]
3. Cayo, A.K.; Yen, T.W.; Misustin, S.M.; Wall, K.; Wilson, S.D.; Evans, D.B.; Wang, T.S. Predicting the need for calcium and calcitriol supplementation after total thyroidectomy: Results of a prospective, randomized study. *Surgery* **2012**, *152*, 1059–1067. [CrossRef] [PubMed]
4. Paduraru, D.N.; Ion, D.; Carsote, M.; Andronic, O.; Bolocan, A. Post-thyroidectomy Hypocalcemia—Risk Factors and Management. *Chirurgia* **2019**, *114*, 564–570. [CrossRef] [PubMed]
5. Thomusch, O.; Machens, A.; Sekulla, C.; Ukkat, J.; Brauckhoff, M.; Dralle, H. The impact of surgical technique on postoperative hypoparathyroidism in bilateral thyroid surgery: A multivariate analysis of 5846 consecutive patients. *Surgery* **2003**, *133*, 180–185. [CrossRef] [PubMed]
6. Bilezikian, J.P.; Khan, A.; Potts, J.T., Jr.; Brandi, M.L.; Clarke, B.L.; Shoback, D.; Juppner, H.; D'Amour, P.; Fox, J.; Rejnmark, L.; et al. Hypoparathyroidism in the adult: Epidemiology, diagnosis, pathophysiology, target-organ involvement, treatment, and challenges for future research. *J. Bone Miner. Res.* **2011**, *26*, 2317–2337. [CrossRef]
7. Chow, T.L.; Choi, C.Y.; Chiu, A.N. Postoperative PTH monitoring of hypocalcemia expedites discharge after thyroidectomy. *Am. J. Otolaryngol.* **2014**, *35*, 736–740. [CrossRef] [PubMed]
8. Kakava, K.; Tournis, S.; Papadakis, G.; Karelas, I.; Stampouloglou, P.; Kassi, E.; Triantafillopoulos, I.; Villiotou, V.; Karatzas, T. Postsurgical Hypoparathyroidism: A Systematic Review. *In Vivo* **2016**, *30*, 171–179.
9. Cusano, N.E.; Anderson, L.; Rubin, M.R.; Silva, B.C.; Costa, A.G.; Irani, D.; Sliney, J., Jr.; Bilezikian, J.P. Recovery of parathyroid hormone secretion and function in postoperative hypoparathyroidism: A case series. *J. Clin. Endocrinol. Metab.* **2013**, *98*, 4285–4290. [CrossRef]
10. Selberherr, A.; Scheuba, C.; Riss, P.; Niederle, B. Postoperative hypoparathyroidism after thyroidectomy: Efficient and cost-effective diagnosis and treatment. *Surgery* **2015**, *157*, 349–353. [CrossRef]
11. Pfleiderer, A.G.; Ahmad, N.; Draper, M.R.; Vrotsou, K.; Smith, W.K. The timing of calcium measurements in helping to predict temporary and permanent hypocalcaemia in patients having completion and total thyroidectomies. *Ann. R. Coll. Surg. Engl.* **2009**, *91*, 140–146. [CrossRef] [PubMed]
12. Asari, R.; Passler, C.; Kaczirek, K.; Scheuba, C.; Niederle, B. Hypoparathyroidism after total thyroidectomy: A prospective study. *Arch. Surg.* **2008**, *143*, 132–137, discussion 138. [CrossRef] [PubMed]
13. Pattou, F.; Combemale, F.; Fabre, S.; Carnaille, B.; Decoulx, M.; Wemeau, J.L.; Racadot, A.; Proye, C. Hypocalcemia following thyroid surgery: Incidence and prediction of outcome. *World J. Surg.* **1998**, *22*, 718–724. [CrossRef] [PubMed]
14. Erbil, Y.; Barbaros, U.; Temel, B.; Turkoglu, U.; Issever, H.; Bozbora, A.; Ozarmagan, S.; Tezelman, S. The impact of age, vitamin D(3) level, and incidental parathyroidectomy on postoperative hypocalcemia after total or near total thyroidectomy. *Am. J. Surg.* **2009**, *197*, 439–446. [CrossRef] [PubMed]
15. Edafe, O.; Antakia, R.; Laskar, N.; Uttley, L.; Balasubramanian, S.P. Systematic review and meta-analysis of predictors of post-thyroidectomy hypocalcaemia. *Br. J. Surg.* **2014**, *101*, 307–320. [CrossRef]
16. DGAV. Thyroid surgery quality assurance registry of the German Association of Surgeons (DGAV); StuDoQ|Thyroid. 2021. Available online: http://www.dgav.de/studoq.html (accessed on 23 November 2021).
17. Allemeyer, E.H.; Kossow, M.S.; Riemann, B.; Hoffmann, M.W. Risk Factors for Permanent Postoperative Hypoparathyreoidism. *Zentralbl. Chir.* **2019**, *145*, 168–175. [CrossRef]
18. Almquist, M.; Hallgrimsson, P.; Nordenstrom, E.; Bergenfelz, A. Prediction of permanent hypoparathyroidism after total thyroidectomy. *World J. Surg.* **2014**, *38*, 2613–2620. [CrossRef]
19. Evans, J.D. *Straightforward Statistics for the Behavioral Sciences*; Brooks/Cole Pub. Co.: Pacific Grove, CA, USA, 1996.
20. Lorente-Poch, L.; Sancho, J.J.; Muñoz-Nova, J.L.; Sánchez-Velázquez, P.; Sitges-Serra, A. Defining the syndromes of parathyroid failure after total thyroidectomy. *Gland Surg.* **2015**, *4*, 82–90. [CrossRef]
21. Sitges-Serra, A. Etiology and Diagnosis of Permanent Hypoparathyroidism after Total Thyroidectomy. *J. Clin. Med.* **2021**, *10*, 543. [CrossRef]
22. Harsløf, T.; Rolighed, L.; Rejnmark, L. Huge variations in definition and reported incidence of postsurgical hypoparathyroidism: A systematic review. *Endocrine* **2019**, *64*, 176–183. [CrossRef]
23. Koimtzis, G.D.; Stefanopoulos, L.; Giannoulis, K.; Papavramidis, T.S. What are the real rates of temporary hypoparathyroidism following thyroidectomy? It is a matter of definition: A systematic review. *Endocrine* **2021**, *73*, 1–7. [CrossRef] [PubMed]
24. Mathur, A.; Nagarajan, N.; Kahan, S.; Schneider, E.B.; Zeiger, M.A. Association of Parathyroid Hormone Level with Postthyroidectomy Hypocalcemia: A Systematic Review. *JAMA Surg.* **2018**, *153*, 69–76. [CrossRef] [PubMed]
25. Strajina, V.; Dy, B.M.; McKenzie, T.J.; Thompson, G.B.; Lyden, M.L. Predicting Postthyroidectomy Hypocalcemia: Improving Predictive Ability of Parathyroid Hormone Level. *Am. Surg.* **2020**, *86*, 121–126. [CrossRef] [PubMed]

26. Suwannasarn, M.; Jongjaroenprasert, W.; Chayangsu, P.; Suvikapakornkul, R.; Sriphrapradang, C. Single measurement of intact parathyroid hormone after thyroidectomy can predict transient and permanent hypoparathyroidism: A prospective study. *Asian J. Surg.* **2017**, *40*, 350–356. [CrossRef]
27. Sitges-Serra, A.; Gomez, J.; Barczynski, M.; Lorente-Poch, L.; Iacobone, M.; Sancho, J. A nomogram to predict the likelihood of permanent hypoparathyroidism after total thyroidectomy based on delayed serum calcium and iPTH measurements. *Gland Surg.* **2017**, *6* (Suppl. S1), S11–S19. [CrossRef]
28. Vaitsi, K.D.; Anagnostis, P.; Veneti, S.; Papavramidis, T.S.; Goulis, D.G. Preoperative Vitamin D Deficiency is a Risk Factor for Postthyroidectomy Hypoparathyroidism: A Systematic Review and Meta-Analysis of Observational Studies. *J. Clin. Endocrinol. Metab.* **2021**, *106*, 1209–1224. [CrossRef]

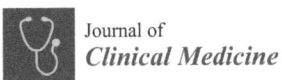

Article

[^{18}F]fluoro-ethylcholine-PET Plus 4D-CT (FEC-PET-CT): A Break-Through Tool to Localize the "Negative" Parathyroid Adenoma. One Year Follow Up Results Involving 170 Patients

Constantin Smaxwil [1,*], Philip Aschoff [2], Gerald Reischl [3,4], Mirjam Busch [1], Joachim Wagner [1], Julia Altmeier [1], Oswald Ploner [5] and Andreas Zielke [1]

1. Department of Endocrine Surgery, Endokrines Zentrum Stuttgart, Diakonie-Klinikum Stuttgart, 70176 Stuttgart, Germany; buschm@diak-stuttgart.de (M.B.); Wagner@diak-stuttgart.de (J.W.); julia.altmeier@diak-stuttgart.de (J.A.); andreas.zielke@diak-stuttgart.de (A.Z.)
2. Department of Nuclear Medicine and PET-CT Centre, Institute of Diagnostic and Interventional Radiology, Diakonie-Klinikum Stuttgart, 70176 Stuttgart, Germany; aschoff@diak-stuttgart.de
3. Department of Preclinical Imaging and Radiopharmacy, Werner Siemens Imaging Center, Eberhard Karls University of Tuebingen, 72076 Tuebingen, Germany; Gerald.Reischl@med.uni-tuebingen.de
4. Cluster of Excellence iFIT (EXC 2180) Image Guided and Functionally Instructed Tumor Therapies, University of Tuebingen, 72076 Tuebingen, Germany
5. Department of Internal Medicine, Endocrinology, Endokrines Zentrum Stuttgart, Diakonie-Klinikum Stuttgart, 70176 Stuttgart, Germany; Ploner@diak-stuttgart.de
* Correspondence: smaxwil@diak-stuttgart.de; Tel.: +49-711-9913301; Fax: +49-711-9913309

Citation: Smaxwil, C.; Aschoff, P.; Reischl, G.; Busch, M.; Wagner, J.; Altmeier, J.; Ploner, O.; Zielke, A. [^{18}F]fluoro-ethylcholine-PET Plus 4D-CT (FEC-PET-CT): A Break-Through Tool to Localize the "Negative" Parathyroid Adenoma. One Year Follow Up Results Involving 170 Patients. *J. Clin. Med.* **2021**, *10*, 1648. https://doi.org/10.3390/jcm10081648

Academic Editor: Marek Ruchala

Received: 17 February 2021
Accepted: 25 March 2021
Published: 13 April 2021

Publisher's Note: MDPI stays neutral with regard to jurisdictional claims in published maps and institutional affiliations.

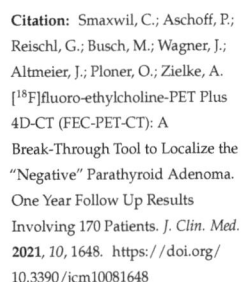

Copyright: © 2021 by the authors. Licensee MDPI, Basel, Switzerland. This article is an open access article distributed under the terms and conditions of the Creative Commons Attribution (CC BY) license (https://creativecommons.org/licenses/by/4.0/).

Abstract: Background: The diagnostic performance of [^{18}F]fluoro-ethylcholine-PET-CT&4D-CT (FEC-PET&4D-CT) to identify parathyroid adenomas (PA) was analyzed when ultrasound (US) or MIBI-Scan (MS) failed to localize. Postsurgical one year follow-up data are presented. Methods: Patients in whom US and MS delivered either incongruent or entirely negative findings were subjected to FEC-PET&4D-CT and cases from July 2017 to June 2020 were analyzed, retrospectively. Cervical exploration with intraoperative PTH-monitoring (IO-PTH) was performed. Imaging results were correlated to intraoperative findings, and short term and one year postoperative follow-up data. Results: From July 2017 to June 2020 in 171 FEC-PET&4D-CTs 159 (92.9%) PAs were suggested. 147 patients already had surgery, FEC-PET&4D-CT accurately localized in 141; false neg. 4, false pos. 2, global sensitivity 0.97; accuracy 0.96, PPV 0.99. All of the 117 patients that already have completed their 12-month postoperative follow up had normal biochemical parameter, i.e., no signs of persisting disease. However, two cases may have a potential for recurrent disease, for a cure rate of at least 98.3%. Conclusion: FEC-PET&4D-CT shows unprecedented results regarding the accuracy localizing PAs. The one-year-follow-up data demonstrate a high cure rate. We, therefore, suggest FEC-PET-CT as the relevant diagnostic tool for the localization of PAs when US fails to localize PA, especially after previous surgery to the neck.

Keywords: parathyroid adenoma; hyperparathyroidism; PET-CT; FEC; FCH

1. Introduction

Primary hyperparathyroidism (pHPT) is the third most common endocrine disorder, with the highest incidence in postmenopausal women. Asymptomatic disease is common and severe disease with renal stones and metabolic bone disease arises less frequently now than it did 20–30 years ago [1]. pHPT is diagnosed by elevated serum calcium and parathyroid hormone (PTH) levels. In about 90% of cases, it is caused by a single parathyroid adenoma (PA) and less often by parathyroid hyperplasia due to multiglandular disease. pHPT can be cured only by surgical removal of the parathyroid adenoma (PA) [2]. Because most patients will only have one PA, they benefit from focused interventions. The success of such "targeted" parathyroid surgery relies on a sensitive and accurate preoperative imaging technique—and an experienced surgeon. The results of focused operations of preoperatively unequivocally localized PA are largely equivalent to a formal, bilateral neck exploration [3]. PAs can be localized by multiple modalities such as high-resolution (7.0–10.0 MHz) ultrasonography (US), computed tomography (CT), magnetic resonance imaging (MRI), and scintigraphy. Parathyroid scintigraphy involves a number of different radiotracers and protocols but [99mTc]Tc-Sestamibi (MS) is the most often used. However, up to one-third of patients with adenomas will be negative with either US or MS [4].

During the last two decades, the role of positron emission tomography/computed tomography (PET/CT) imaging using specific PET tracers has been highlighted. Several PET radiotracers have been introduced for the assessment of pHPT. One of the more commonly used is [^{11}C]methionine. Recently, the feasibility of [^{18}F]fluorocholine (FCH) and [^{18}F]fluoro-ethylcholine (FEC) to localize PAs has been initially reported in case reports and small case-series, but its broader application was recently presented in a clinical study involving 139 operated patients [5]. Most of these reports focused primarily on the degree of agreement between preoperative imaging and intraoperative findings and highlighted the diagnostic parameter. However, most of these studies have not present long term cure rates, hence the clinical utility of FEC/FCH-PET-CT as a diagnostic tool for the localization of PA has yet to be determined.

Here, we present data of a consecutive series of patients who had [^{18}F]fluoro-ethylcholine-PET-CT plus 4D-CT (FEC-PET&4D-CT) to localize PA(s) in biochemically proven pHPT when either ultrasound (US) or MIBI-Scan (MS) failed to localize. Moreover, and for the first time, postsurgical one-year follow up data are presented allowing for an assessment of the clinical utility of this new imaging tool.

2. Materials and Methods

2.1. Study Population

Between July 2017 and June 2020, FEC-PET&4D-CT was employed in patients with biochemically proven pHPT in whom US and MS delivered either incongruent or entirely negative findings. Patients that had concordant results during US and MIBI and, thus, double localized PAs were not included into this study. Irrespective of the findings of any of the imaging tools, all patients were offered cervical explorations with intraoperative PTH-monitoring (IO-PTH) and enrolled into our centers structured postoperative follow up program, to determine the short as well as long term results of cervical exploration.

2.2. Preparation of [^{18}F]Fluoro-Ethylcholine (FEC)

For synthesis of FEC for human application, the method of Hara et al. [6] was improved and adopted to a TRACERlab FX$_{F-N}$ automated system (GE Healthcare, Münster, Germany) in a certified GMP environment. Briefly, [^{18}F]fluoride was produced at a PETtrace cyclotron (GE Healthcare, Uppsala, Sweden) and trapped on an anion exchange cartridge (Waters, Milford, MA, USA). Subsequently, radioactivity was eluted and azeotropically dried in presence of Kryptofix 2.2.2 (Merck, Darmstadt, Germany). In a first step, labelling of 1.2-bis(tosyloxy)ethane (Aldrich, Taufkirchen, Germany) with [^{18}F]fluoride/[K/2.2.2] in acetonitrile yielded 2-[^{18}F]fluoro-ethyltosylate, which was purified by HPLC and reversed phase solid phase extraction (RP SPE, Waters, Milford, MA, USA). In a second step, by reaction of the labelled tosylate with N,N-dimethylaminoethanol (DMAE) and subsequent cation exchange SPE (Waters, Milford, MA, USA) purification, FEC was obtained within 55 min, overall. After sterile filtration product volume was ca. 10 mL in buffered saline. Radiopharmaceutical quality control was performed following European Pharmacopoeia (Ph. Eur.) rules. Purity, pH, endotoxin content and sterility met the requirements for parenteralia.

2.3. PET/CT Technique

PET/CT examinations were performed on a Discovery 600—PET/CT-Scanner (GE Healthcare, Milwaukee, WIS, USA). One hour after intravenous administration of 200 MBq of FEC. A nonenhanced CT scan preceded the PET acquisition and was used for attenuation correction. The PET acquisition covered the neck and the chest from the angle of the mandible to the diaphragm (static acquisition, 2 to 3 bed positions, 4 min per bed position) [7]. Subsequently the contrast enhanced CT scans were acquired, comprising a scan in arterial phase with bolus tracking technique and a scan in venous phase with a delay of 80 s [8]. CT and PET images were reconstructed using iterative algorithms (ASiR and SharpIR respectively). For quantitative PET assessment, SUVmax of lesions was recorded.

2.4. Parathyroidectomy

Patients underwent guided, focused minimal invasive parathyroidectomy with intraoperative neuromonitoring and intraoperative PTH-assay (IO-I-PTH, future diagnostics, 6603 BN Wijchen, The Netherlands) following standards set forth by current guidelines [9,10]. In the case of multiglandular disease, a standardized bilateral exploration of the neck was performed.

All individuals included in this series underwent surgery at a high-volume center of reference for thyroid and parathyroid surgery, certified by the German Association of Surgery (DGAV) [11]. All operations were done by one of 5 certified endocrine surgeons, using standardized techniques with a focus to apply minimal invasive techniques whenever possible. These techniques do not mandate extended dissection to visualize all four parathyroid glands if the enlarged gland is readily exposed and intraoperative PTH testing is indicative of biochemical cure.

2.5. Postsurgical Follow up Data

All patients in this series were subject to a standardized perioperative protocol, ensuring biochemical testing for fasting (total serum) calcium and PTH levels between 7 and 8 a.m. on post-operative day (POD) 1 and POD2 as well as POD3 in the rare event, a patient had not yet been discharged. After discharge from the hospital patients were subject to a detailed follow-up program. All patients were followed for at least 12 months postoperatively. To this end, the Endocrine Centers Outcomes Research Unit used structured telephone interviews to assess current medication, laboratory parameter and symptoms of hypo- or hypercalcemia. For the purpose of this analysis, all imaging results (US, MS, FEC-PET-CT, 4D-CT) were correlated to intraoperative findings, histopathology, short term biochemical outcome (i.e., until discharge) as well as the biochemical follow-up data after 12 months.

To accurately determine the post-surgical cure rate of pHPT it is paramount to obtain biochemical parameter 12 months postoperatively. Historically, the terminology of persisting pHPT has been used for cases in whom biochemical cure is registered only for brief periods, e.g., less than 12–24 weeks, and recurrent pHPT is diagnosed in individuals in whom calcium and PTH have remained within the normal range for periods of more than 3 but less than 12 months [12–17]. Hence, in this study biochemical parameter were addressed at 12 months post-surgery to determine the cure rate. In accordance with guidelines, entirely normal values of total serum calcium and PTH were registered as "cure", whereas elevated total serum calcium above the upper limit of norm concurred by elevated levels of PTH above the upper limit of norm were defined biochemical signs of persisting pHPT. Likewise, simultaneously elevated levels of calcium and PTH, albeit within the normal range, were defined "potential recurrence" and, thus, potential failure.

2.6. Handling of Data and Analysis; Definition of Diagnostic Accuracy

All data were prospectively documented as individual perioperative datasets using the hyperparathyroidism-module of the StuDoQ-quality assurance registry of the German Surgical Association (DGAV) [11]. All data computed for this publication were pseudonymized or aggregate non-individual data. There were no missing values. Descriptive statistic was used to summarize patients' characteristics retrospectively. Continuous variables are reported as mean and standard deviation (SD) including 95% confidence interval and are compared between groups using two-sample independent t-tests. Categorical variables are summarized as frequencies (%). Results of the localization of a PA by FEC-PET-CTs were recorded as follows: surgical removal of a PA at the site predicted by FEC-PET-CT followed by an adequate drop of intraoperative PTH level as well as histopathological confirmation of the PA (i.e., confirmed PA) was recorded as a true positive result. Likewise, surgical removal of a confirmed PA at a site different from the one predicted by FEC-PET-CT was recorded as a false positive result and detection of a confirmed PA in a case where FEC-PET-CT had been non-diagnostic, was recorded as a false negative result.

2.7. Ethics Approval and Consent to Participate

This study was approved by the Institutional Review Board of the Diakonie-Klinikum Stuttgart and conducted in cooperation with the Endocrine Centers certified Outcomes Research Unit. All methods were carried out in accordance with the Declaration of Helsinki and the approved guidelines. The data enrolled in this study were obtained from the centers pseudonymized quality assurance database (StuDoQ, a quality assurance database for certified centers of Endocrine Surgery of the German Association of Surgeons, DGAV [11]). Ethical committees determined that the data presented in this article do not represent a human participant research study, do not include personal identifying information, and were carried out for the reason of quality monitoring and assurance. Therefore, this analysis did not require informed consent other than the consent obtained prior to entering data into the StuDoQ Database. However, prior to entering data into the StuDoQ database, all patients gave informed consent, both with regard to FEC-imaging as well as disease specific data acquisition and secondary analysis into the StuDoQ Registry.

3. Results

3.1. Patient Characteristics

From July 2017 to June 02020, 454 patients were operated for pHPT at our department (64 with prior surgery to the neck (14.1%) including 18 redo-for-HPT (4%)). During this period 171 FEC-PET-CTs were performed. Of these, 152 were performed in combination with 4D-CT (88.9%), in 19 patients no contrast enhanced 4D-CT was performed due to hyperthyroidism or renal dysfunction. Most of the patients had FEC-PET-CT&4D-CT either because of incongruent (48.0%) or entirely negative imaging results (43.3%) by US and/or MS. Nine patients (5.2%) had a negative US without MS performed, and six patients (4.2%) were positive on US and MS but still received FEC-PET-CTs with 4D-CT to confirm the localization because of extensive previous neck surgery. A total of 137 of the 171 patients (80.1%) were female, and 44 were redo-cases (25.8%) either after previous thyroid ($n = 27$, 15.8%) or parathyroid surgery ($n = 17$, 10.0%). All patients had preoperative clearly elevated Calcium (mean 2.78 ± 0.17 mmol/L (2.76–2.81; 95% confidence interval, CI) and elevated PTH (124.6 ± 66.7 ng/L (CI 114.6–134.6). Noticeable was a significant ($p = 0.02$) higher PTH-level and even more significant ($p = 0.001$) higher Calcium-level in patients with previous parathyroid surgery as compared to patients without previous surgery (Table 1).

Table 1. Patients characteristics of 171 FEC-PET-CT&4D-CT from July 2017 to June 2020 for all patients and the two subgroups with previous thyroid and parathyroid surgery. Qualitative data are expressed as numbers; continuous data are expressed as mean ± SD and 95% confidence interval. Reference range Calcium: 2.2–2.6 mmol/L; PTH 12–45 ng/L. * $p < 0.05$ and † $p = 0.001$ as compared to patients without previous surgery.

Patient Characteristics			
	All	Prev. Thyroid Proc.	Prev. Parathyroid Proc.
Number (%)	171 (100%)	27 (15.8%)	17 (10.0%)
Sex			
Male	34 (19.9%)	4 (14.8%)	4 (23.5%)
Female	137 (80.1%)	23 (85.2%)	13 (76.5%)
Age (years)	61.5 ± 12.8 (59.5–63.4)	66.1 ± 9.6 (62.5–69.8)	57.0 ± 15.2 (49.7–64.2)
Biochemistry			
Calcium	2.78 ± 0.17 (2.76–2.81)	2.77 ± 0.15 (2.71–2.82)	2.88 ± 0.22 (2.77–2.98) †
PTH	124.6 ± 66.9 (114.6–134.6)	129.4 ± 56.3 (108.1–150.6)	180.1 ± 115.3 (125.2–234.9) *

3.2. Localization of PA by Ultrasound, MIBI-Scintigraphy and FEC-PET-CT plus 4D-CT

Overall, FEC-PET-CT with 4D-CT resulted in findings suggestive of a potential PA in 159 patients (93.0%). Of these 171 patients, preoperative diagnostic work up recorded 109 (63.7%) individuals to have been nondiagnostic (negative) on cervical US and 74 (43.3%) were also MS negative; these individuals were thus "double negative" for both US and MIBI. Of the 109 US negative patients FEC-PET&4D-CT suggested a PA in 98 (89.9%) and of the 62 US positive patients in 61 (98.4%) patients.

Of the 74 patients in whom US and MS did not offer a localization of a PA (double negative) FEC-PET&4D-CT suggested a PA in 66 (89.2%) patients.

A total of 26 patients had a positive finding during MIBI-scintigraphy (MS) but were negative on US and a further 9 cases that were negative on US had not undergone MS. Of these 35 patients FEC-PET&4D-CT suggested a PA in 29 (82.9%) patients.

There were 44 patients with previous surgery to either the thyroid or the parathyroid glands. Twelve out of these 44 patients with congruent findings during US and MS still received FEC-PET&4D-CT—mainly because of the extent of preoperative surgery or to rule out parathyreomatosis. In this subset of 44 patients requiring secondary surgery, localization of PA was feasible in all but one, for a detection rate of 97.7% (Table 2).

Table 2. Absolute numbers and percentage of patients with positive and negative localization of a parathyroid adenoma in the preoperative work-up for all patients and subgroups with either previous thyroid or parathyroid surgery and the respective number of positive findings in FEC-PET-CT&4D-CT.

Results of Preoperative Ultrasound (US) and Mibi-Scan (MS) Localization			
	All	Prev. Thyroid pProc.	Prev. Parathyroid Proc.
n	171	27	17
US negative	109 (63.7%)	16 (59.3%)	11 (64.7%)
and MS negative	74 (43.3%)	9 (33.3%)	9 (52.9%)
and MS positive	26 (15.2%)	7 (26.0%)	2 (11.8%)
and MS not done	9 (5.3%)	-	-
FEC-Pet-CT&4D-CT pos	94 (86.2%)	16 (100%)	10 (90.9%)
US positive	62 (26.3%)	11 (40.7%)	6 (35.3%)
and MS negative	57 (33.3%)	9 (33.3%)	4 (23.5%)
and MS positive	3 (1.8%)	1 (3.7%)	2 (11.8%)
and MS not done	2 (1.2%)	1 (3.7%)	-
FEC-Pet-CT&4D-CT pos	61 (98.4%)	11 (100%)	6 (100%)

An example of the imaging resolution of FEC-PET-CT is given in Figure 1, of a patient with recurrent pHPT 18 years after initial surgery for pHPT. The reason for recurrence was a parathyroid spillage parathyreomatosis caused by the primary operation on the left side of the neck. However, FEC-PET-CT demonstrated a discernible FEC-retention next to a clip in the sternocleidoid muscle, revealing a tiny amount of autotransplanted parathyroid tissue (Figure 1). Another example is given in Figure 2 of a patient who had total thyroidectomy and local lymphnode clearance because of thyroid cancer and was diagnosed to have pHPT. This patient had been "double negative" on US and MS during preoperative workup. The prima facie demonstration of the left upper descended parathyroid gland made it possible to choose a focused lateral approach to remove the PA. Because of severe pre-existing conditions (ASA IV: acute on chronic renal failure, severe arterial hypertension, exacerbated COPD, and chronic depression) and because of the pin-pointed localization the procedure was done under local anesthesia in this patient.

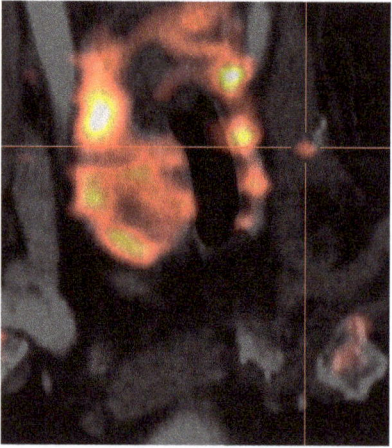

Figure 1. Autotransplanted tissue of a parathyroid adenoma, 18 years after initial surgery depicted by FEC-PET-CT-scan and localized into the left sternocleidoid muscle next to a clip. To the right of the trachea, the right thyroid lobe is seen and to the left of the trachea a chain of parathyroid adenomata, caused by parathyreomatosis is noted.

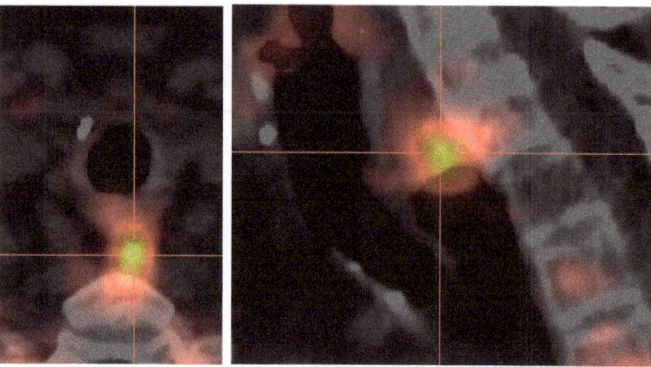

Figure 2. a+b Parathyroid adenoma (PA) of the descended upper left gland in a patient who had total thyroidectomy and central lymph node dissection because of thyroid cancer 10 years earlier.

3.3. Degree of Intraoperative Agreement and Postoperative Long-Term Results

147 of the 171 patients of this cohort already had surgery, including 25 with previous thyroid and 14 with previous parathyroid procedures. The patient's characteristics of this subset of patients showed no difference to the entire group of patients. Similar to the entire cohort, levels of calcium and PTH were higher in patients with previous parathyroid surgery as compared to patients after thyroid or without previous surgery to the neck.

Of all operated patients FEC-PET-CT plus 4D-CT accurately localized PA(s) to the respective side of the neck in 141 patients; it was found to have been false negative in four and false positive in two patients, respectively, for a global sensitivity of 0.97; accuracy of 0.96 and PPV of 0.99.

FEC-PET-CT successfully localized the PA in 140 of 147 patients, and in all of the patients that had previous surgery to the neck it correctly predicted the site of the PA. We found neither significant difference in SUV nor the size of the PA in the FEC-PET-CT and no difference in the postoperative PTH-decrease for all patients compared to patients after previous surgery. Pathological findings of parathyreomatosis were only demonstrated in the group with previous parathyroid surgery (Table 3).

With regard to the side effects of surgery two patients were treated for postoperative bleeding—one patient had undergone synchronous thyroidectomy for Graves' Disease and one was a reoperative case for persisting pHPT. There were two cases of temporary vocal cord dysfunction. One patient with previous thyroid resection had a vocal cord paresis contralateral to the current operated side. Another patient had a paresis after a combined procedure involving a simultaneous thyroid lobectomy. Both patients had full recovery of their vocal cord function within six months after surgery, respectively.

Table 3. Patients' characteristics, intraoperative agreement (of preoperative FEC-PET-CT localized parathyroid adenomas) and postoperative results of patients operated after imaging with FEC-PET-CT. Data are presented from the entire cohort of 147 patients and the subgroups with previous thyroid and parathyroid surgery. Qualitative data are expressed as numbers; continuous data as mean ± SD and 95% confidence interval. * One patient with previous thyroid resection developed a vocal cord paresis contralateral to the current operated side and another paresis occurred ipsilateral in a patient with simultaneous hemithyroidectomy. ** One patient had synchronous thyroidectomy for Graves' Disease, and another had a reoperation for persisting pHPT, respectively (Ref. range Calcium 2.2–2.6 mmol/L; PTH 15–65 ng/L).

	Degree of Intraoperative Agreement and Postoperative Results		
	All Operated Patients	Prev. Thyroid Proc.	Prev. Parathyroid Proc.
	147	25	14
Female	119 (81.0%)	22 (88%)	11 (78.6%)
Age (y)	60.8 ± 8.1 (56.8–65.0)	65.4 ± 9.6 (61.6–69.2)	56.9 ± 15.6 (48.7–65.0)
BMI	26.8 ± 3.8 (23.5–30.1)	27.0 ± 5.1 (24.9–29.2)	27.3 ± 3.5 (25.1–29.4)
preop biochemistry			
Calcium (total, mmol/L)	2.79 ± 0.13 (2.72–2.85)	2.78 ± 0.15 (2.72–2.84)	2.92 ± 0.19 (2.82–3.02)
PTH (ng/L)	129.0 ± 58.1 (99.6–158.4)	131.0 ± 58.3 (108.1–153.8)	199.9 ± 117.7 (138.2–231.5)
FEC-PET CT			
pos for PA	140 (95.2%)	25 (100%)	14 (100%)
neg for PA	7 (4.8%)	-	-
size of the PA (mm)	11.0 ± 5.8 (8.1–13.9)	10.8 ± 4.2 (9.1–12.4)	13.7 ± 10.4 (8.3–19.1)
SUV	5.3 ± 1.9 (4.4–6.3)	5.5 ± 2.3 (4.6–6.4)	5.5 ± 2.7 (4.1–6.9)

Table 3. Cont.

	Degree of Intraoperative Agreement and Postoperative Results		
	All Operated Patients	Prev. Thyroid Proc.	Prev. Parathyroid Proc.
Histology			
single adenoma	136 (92.5%)	23 (92.0%)	11 (78.6%)
double adenoma	5 (3.4%)	2 (8.0%)	1 (7.1%)
hyperplasia	3 (2.0%)	-	-
parathyreomatosis	2 (1.4%)	-	2 (14.3%)
normal parathyroid gland	1 (0.7%)	-	-
postoperative data			
PTH (ng/L)	26.2 ± 15.1 (18.6–33.9)	24.6 ± 12.9 (19.2–30.0)	31.4 ± 26.9 (16.8–46.1)
Paresis of vocal cord *	2 (1.4%)	1 (4.0%)	-
Postoperative bleeding **	2 (1.4%)	-	1 (7.1%)

The rate of persisting HPT in this series was zero since none of the 117 patients that already have completed their 12-month postoperative follow up had biochemical signs of persistent disease. However, two cases (one case of recurrent pHPT who had repeat surgery for PA 18 years after the primary procedure and one case of pHPT with removal of a solitary PA) had elevated levels of both PTH and Calcium, albeit well within the normal range. Taking account of these two patients, which may have a potential for recurrent disease in the future, the overall cure rate would amount to 115 of 117 cases (98.3%). The cure rate (Table 4) of the subset of double negative patients would amount to at least 49 of 50 (98.0%) and the cure rate of patients with previous surgery to the thyroid and parathyroid to at least 26 of 27 (96.3%).

Table 4. Twelve months biochemical follow up data and cure rate of patients operated after imaging with FEC-PET-CT. Data are presented from the entire cohort of 147 patients enrolled between July 2017 and June 2020 and the subgroups with previous thyroid and parathyroid surgery. Qualitative data are expressed as numbers; continuous data as mean ± SD and 95% confidence interval. Ref. range Calcium 2.2–2.6 mmol/L; PTH 15–65 ng/L) * US and MS negative PAs.

	One Year Follow Up Results		
12 Months Follow Up Data	All Operated Patients	Double Neg. *	Prev. Neck Surgery
	117	50	27
PTH (ng/L)	44.3 ± 18.4 (40.6–48.0)	44.5 ± 17.9 (38.9–50.0)	48.9 ± 18.0 (39.5–58.3)
Ca (total, mmol/L)	2.37 ± 0.13 (2.35–2.39)	2.37 ± 0.13 (2.33–2.41)	2.36 ± 0.15 (2.24–2.44)
Paresis of vocal cord	-	-	-
Cure rate (at least)	115 (98.3%)	49 (98%)	26 (96.3%)

4. Discussion

Historically, bilateral surgical exploration of the neck using surgical protocols that explore all of the possible sites of PA have produced excellent clinical outcome in experienced hands. Over the past two decades there has been a shift towards minimally invasive parathyroidectomy (MIP); a focused operation whereby only the affected PA is removed. Compared to bilateral neck exploration, MIP is associated with smaller incisions, shorter operating time, lower complication rates and faster recovery from postoperative hypoparathyroidism [18,19]. Focused operations, however, rely on preoperative localization of the PA as well as intraoperative PTH-monitoring [9].

There are a number of modalities for preoperative localization such as Ultrasound (US), MIBI-scintigraphy (MS), PET-CT, MRI as well as fine-needle aspiration with measurement of PTH. The most recent guideline (NICE 2019) recommends cervical US and suggests a second modality, such as MS, if it will further guide the surgical approach [20]. Likewise, the American Association of Endocrine Surgeons (AAES) guideline recommends US and another "high-resolution imaging" for operative planning of focused operations [9]. Adherence to these protocols results in favorable clinical outcome: a recent study on 682 patients with pHPT from a tertiary referral center, reported an overall one year cure rate of 97.4% and of 87.5% in the setting of surgery for persisting disease [21].

A recent meta-analysis underscored the utility of US as the first-line tool for the detection of PAs with a pooled sensitivity of 76.1% (95% CI 70.4–81.4%) and positive predictive value (PPV) of 93.2% (90.7–95.3%), respectively [22]. MS had a pooled sensitivity of 78.9% (64–90.6%) and PPV of 90.7% (83.5–96.0%) [23]. In the 20% of cases in whom either or both of these methods fail to localize, PET-CT with [11C]methionine is most often employed. 11C has a half-life of only 20 min, which requires on-site production rendering it unfit for wide-spread use [24]. Using FCH, with the longer-lived 18F (half-life ca. 110 min) the need for an on-site cyclotron is obviated. FCH has only recently been used for the localization of PA in a small number of studies. However, the results have been very encouraging [25].

In this study the rate by which PAs are localized by FEC-PET-CT that had not been detected by US and MS, was found to be well above 90%, and the rate of detection in patients with previous surgery to the neck including reoperations for pHPT was above 90%, too. Our findings are, therefore, consistent with those of other case series [26]. Moreover, and for the first time, this study delivers one year follow up data, confirming a global cure rate for PAs localized by FEC-PET of at least 98.3% and at least 96.3% for PA not localized with US and MS. The clinical utility of FEC-PET-CT is underscored by a cure rate of 100% for patients with previous surgery to the neck including failed parathyroid procedures. Although the number of patients with persisting and recurrent pHPT in this study was only 16, it would still appear, that the use of this novel imaging modality may allow to obtain a control of hypercalcemia more often than has been reported before [14].

Because FCH-PET-CT causes less radiation exposure in comparison to MS [27] and taking account of its impressive diagnostic performance, a recent review already suggested FCH as the one and only "one-stop-shop" imaging modality [24]. US, however, has no radiation exposure and was shown to be a very cost-effective tool (21). Therefore, it is unlikely to be replaced as the first line imaging tool. This is underscored by the results of this current study, where all of the PAs demonstrated by US were confirmed by FEC and—more importantly—also, at the time of surgery. This would suggest the greatest clinical utility of FEC to be found in patients with a negative finding on US.

There are some limitations in this study for critical discussion. As this is a retrospective study, the criteria as to when FEC-PET-CT was performed were not stringent. It is for this reason, that we analyzed the subgroup of cases where the PA was not localized during US and MS. This is a well-defined set of patients in whom additional diagnostic is consented by guidelines, and the results obtained in this subset were comparable to those of the entire cohort.

Another weakness of this study is that some of the patients with FEC-PET-CT have yet to undergo surgery or complete their one year follow up, and, finally, this study did not evaluate the relationship between the success rate of PET-CT and the exact anatomical location of the PA, the size or weight of the specimen removed or the extent of the surgical procedure. At this time, and given the surprisingly small number of PA missed by FEC-PET-CT, we believe, that the analysis of failure of FEC will be feasible as soon as larger data sets from quality assurance registries such as the StuDoQ register become available [11]. Moreover, a protocol for a prospective randomized trial has just been published [28].

Finally, in this cohort of diagnostically challenging patients we used FEC always in combination with 4D-CT, which many consider the current gold-standard diagnostic tool. Because these patients had been preselected for negative US and/or MS, a comparative analysis of the diagnostic effect of either of these tools is therefore not feasible. However, when we decided to add FEC to our escalating protocol of diagnostic procedures, there were no data to expect FEC to stand out with such robust diagnostic performance. Keeping this result in mind, further prospective studies may be warranted, comparing the diagnostic performance of 4DCT and FEC as upfront diagnostic tools.

Despite these limitations, we believe this study has shown that FEC-PET-CT&4D-CT delivers unprecedented results regarding the accuracy by which PAs are localized. This was especially true in clinically challenging scenarios as well as reoperative cases. FEC-PET-CT allowed for focused as opposed to bilateral cervical explorations in almost all of the cases and had a very favorable one-year cure rate.

We therefore consider FEC-PET-CT to be the imaging method of choice for the localization of PAs when US failed to localize the PA, and that it may be particularly helpful to localize PA in patients that already had previous surgery to the thyroid or parathyroid.

Author Contributions: Conceptualization, C.S., P.A., O.P., and A.Z.; methodology, C.S. and P.A.; software, C.S.; validation, C.S. and A.Z.; radioisotope investigation, G.R.; resources, M.B. and J.W.; data curation, C.S. and J.A.; writing—original draft preparation, C.S. and A.Z.; writing—final review and editing, C.S., P.A., G.R., M.B., and O.P.; visualization, M.B. and J.A. All authors have read and agreed to the published version of the manuscript.

Funding: This research received no external funding.

Institutional Review Board Statement: This study was approved by the Institutional Review Board of the Diakonie-Klinikum Stuttgart and conducted by the Endocrine Centers certified Outcomes Research Unit. All methods were carried out in accordance with the Declaration of Helsinki and the approved guidelines. The data enrolled in this study were obtained from the centers pseudonymized quality assurance database (since 2017 the StuDoQ-Database for certified centers of Endocrine Surgery of the German Association of Surgeons, DGAVC).

Informed Consent Statement: Ethical committees determined that the data presented in this article do not represent a human participant research study, do not include personal identifying information, and were carried out in accordance with the relevant legislation for the purpose of quality monitoring and quality assurance. Therefore, this analysis did not require informed consent other than the consent obtained prior to entering data into the StuDoQ Database.

Data Availability Statement: Restrictions apply to the data presented in this study. Data were obtained from the StuDoQ Thyroid Quality Assurance Registry of the German Association of Surgeons (DGAVC) and may be available to third parties only upon request to the SAVC/DGAVC and decision at the discretion of the DGAVC.

Conflicts of Interest: The authors declare no conflict of interest.

Abbreviations

CT	computed tomography
FEC-PET-CT&4D-CT	[^{18}F]fluoro-ethylcholine-PET-CT plus 4D-CT
IO-PTH	intraoperative monitoring of parathyroid hormone
MIP	minimally invasive parathyroidectomy
MRI	magnetic resonance imaging
MS	[^{99m}Tc]Tc-sestamibi scintigraphy
PA	parathyroid adenoma
PET	positron emission tomography
pHPT	primary hyperparathyroidism
POD	post-operative day
PTH	parathyroid hormone
StuDoQ	Thyroid surgery quality assurance registry of the German Association of Surgeons; StuDoQ | Thyroid
SUV	Standard Uptake Value
US	ultrasound
VC	vocal cord
VCP	vocal cord paresis

References

1. Fraser, W.D. Hyperparathyroidism. *Lancet* **2009**, *374*, 145–158. [CrossRef]
2. Weber, T.; Eberle, J.; Messelhäuser, U.; Schiffmann, L.; Nies, C.; Schabram, J.; Zielke, A.; Holzer, K.; Rottler, E.; Henne-Bruns, D.; et al. Parathyroidectomy, elevated depression scores, and suicidal ideation in patients with primary hyperparathyroidism: Results of a prospective multicenter study. *JAMA Surg.* **2013**, *148*, 109–115. [CrossRef]
3. Palazzo, F.F.; Delbridge, L.W. Minimal-access/minimally invasive parathyroidectomy for primary hyperparathyroidism. *Surg. Clin. N. Am.* **2004**, *84*, 717–734. [CrossRef]
4. Prabhu, M.; Damle, N.A. Fluorocholine PET Imaging of Parathyroid Disease. *Indian J. Endocrinol. Metab.* **2018**, *22*, 535–541. [CrossRef]
5. Hocevar, M.; Lezaic, L.; Rep, S.; Zaletel, K.; Kocjan, T.; Sever, M.J.; Zgajnar, J.; Peric, B. Focused parathyroidectomy without intraoperative parathormone testing is safe after pre-operative localization with (18)F-Fluorocholine PET/CT. *Eur. J. Surg. Oncol.* **2017**, *43*, 133–137. [CrossRef]
6. Hara, T.; Kosaka, N.; Kishi, H. Development of (^{18}F)-fluoroethylcholine for cancer imaging with PET: Synthesis, biochemistry, and prostate cancer imaging. *J. Nucl. Med.* **2002**, *43*, 187–199.
7. Michaud, L.; Balogova, S.; Burgess, A.; Ohnona, J.; Huchet, V.; Kerrou, K.; Lefevre, M.; Tassart, M.; Montravers, F.; Perie, S.; et al. A Pilot Comparison of 18F-fluorocholine PET/CT, Ultrasonography and 123I/99mTc-sestaMIBI Dual-Phase Dual-Isotope Scintigraphy in the Preoperative Localization of Hyperfunctioning Parathyroid Glands in Primary or Secondary Hyperparathyroidism: Influence of Thyroid Anomalies. *Medicine (Baltimore)* **2015**, *94*, e1701. [CrossRef]
8. Hoang, J.K.; Sung, W.K.; Bahl, M.; Phillips, C.D. How to perform parathyroid 4D CT: Tips and traps for technique and interpretation. *Radiology* **2014**, *270*, 15–24. [CrossRef] [PubMed]
9. Wilhelm, S.M.; Wang, T.S.; Ruan, D.T.; Lee, J.A.; Asa, S.L.; Duh, Q.Y.; Doherty, G.M.; Herrera, M.F.; Pasieka, J.L.; Perrier, N.D.; et al. The American Association of Endocrine Surgeons Guidelines for Definitive Management of Primary Hyperparathyroidism. *JAMA Surg.* **2016**, *151*, 959–968. [CrossRef]
10. CAEK. S2k-Leitlinie HPT: Chirurgisches Management des Primären und Renalen Hyperparathyreoidismus. AWMF (Currently under Revision). 2021. Available online: https://www.awmf.org/leitlinien/detail/ll/174-006.html (accessed on 30 March 2021).
11. DGAV. Thyroid Surgery Quality Assurance Registry of the German Association of Surgeons (DGAV); StuDoQ|Thyroid. Available online: http://www.dgav.de/studoq.html (accessed on 30 March 2021).
12. Guerin, C.; Paladino, N.C.; Lowery, A.; Castinetti, F.; Taieb, D.; Sebag, F. Persistent and recurrent hyperparathyroidism. *Updates Surg.* **2017**, *69*, 161–169. [CrossRef] [PubMed]
13. Clark, O.H.; Way, L.W.; Hunt, T.K. Recurrent hyperparathyroidism. *Ann. Surg.* **1976**, *184*, 391–402. [CrossRef]
14. Karakas, E.; Zielke, A.; Dietz, C.; Rothmund, M. Reoperation for primary hyperparathyroidism. *Chirurg* **2005**, *76*, 207–216. [CrossRef]
15. Mundschenk, J.; Klose, S.; Lorenz, K.; Dralle, H.; Lehnert, H. Diagnostic strategies and surgical procedures in persistent or recurrent primary hyperparathyroidism. *Exp. Clin. Endocrinol. Diabetes* **1999**, *107*, 331–336. [CrossRef] [PubMed]
16. Allemeyer, E.H.; Kossow, M.S.; Riemann, B.; Hoffmann, M.W. Risk Factors for Permanent Postoperative Hypoparathyroidism. *Zentralbl. Chir.* **2020**, *145*, 168–175. [CrossRef]
17. Al-Dhahri, S.F.; Mubasher, M.; Mufarji, K.; Allam, O.S.; Terkawi, A.S. Factors predicting post-thyroidectomy hypoparathyroidism recovery. *World J. Surg.* **2014**, *38*, 2304–2310. [CrossRef]
18. Sackett, W.R.; Barraclough, B.; Reeve, T.S.; Delbridge, L.W. Worldwide trends in the surgical treatment of primary hyperparathyroidism in the era of minimally invasive parathyroidectomy. *Arch. Surg.* **2002**, *137*, 1055–1059. [CrossRef] [PubMed]
19. Irvin, G.L., 3rd; Carneiro, D.M.; Solorzano, C.C. Progress in the operative management of sporadic primary hyperparathyroidism over 34 years. *Ann. Surg.* **2004**, *239*, 704–708, discussion 708–711. [CrossRef]
20. [NG132], N.g. Hyperparathyroidism (Primary): Diagnosis, Assessment and Initial Management. Available online: https://www.nice.org.uk/guidance/ng132/chapter/Recommendations (accessed on 30 March 2021).
21. Dillenberger, S.; Bartsch, D.K.; Maurer, E.; Kann, P.H. Single Centre Experience in Patients with Primary Hyperparathyroidism: Sporadic, Lithium-associated and in Multiple Endocrine Neoplasia. *Exp. Clin. Endocrinol. Diabetes* **2020**, *128*, 693–698. [CrossRef]
22. Cheung, K.; Wang, T.S.; Farrokhyar, F.; Roman, S.A.; Sosa, J.A. A meta-analysis of preoperative localization techniques for patients with primary hyperparathyroidism. *Ann. Surg. Oncol.* **2012**, *19*, 577–583. [CrossRef]
23. Lubitz, C.C.; Stephen, A.E.; Hodin, R.A.; Pandharipande, P. Preoperative localization strategies for primary hyperparathyroidism: An economic analysis. *Ann. Surg. Oncol.* **2012**, *19*, 4202–4209. [CrossRef]
24. Giovanella, L.; Bacigalupo, L.; Treglia, G.; Piccardo, A. Will (18)F-choline PET/CT replace other methods of preoperative parathyroid imaging? *Endocrine* **2020**, *71*, 285–297. [CrossRef]
25. Cuderman, A.; Senica, K.; Rep, S.; Hocevar, M.; Kocjan, T.; Sever, M.J.; Zaletel, K.; Lezaic, L. (18)F-Fluorocholine PET/CT in Primary Hyperparathyroidism: Superior Diagnostic Performance to Conventional Scintigraphic Imaging for Localization of Hyperfunctioning Parathyroid Glands. *J. Nucl. Med.* **2020**, *61*, 577–583. [CrossRef]
26. Broos, W.A.M.; Wondergem, M.; Knol, R.J.J.; van der Zant, F.M. Parathyroid imaging with (18)F-fluorocholine PET/CT as a first-line imaging modality in primary hyperparathyroidism: A retrospective cohort study. *EJNMMI Res.* **2019**, *9*, 72. [CrossRef] [PubMed]

27. Rep, S.; Hocevar, M.; Vaupotic, J.; Zdesar, U.; Zaletel, K.; Lezaic, L. (18)F-choline PET/CT for parathyroid scintigraphy: Significantly lower radiation exposure of patients in comparison to conventional nuclear medicine imaging approaches. *J. Radiol. Prot.* **2018**, *38*, 343–356. [CrossRef] [PubMed]
28. Quak, E.; Lasne Cardon, A.; Ciappuccini, R.; Lasnon, C.; Bastit, V.; Le Henaff, V.; Lireux, B.; Foucras, G.; Jaudet, C.; Berchi, C.; et al. Upfront F18-choline PET/CT versus Tc99m-sestaMIBI SPECT/CT guided surgery in primary hyperparathyroidism: The randomized phase III diagnostic trial APACH2. *BMC Endocr. Disord.* **2021**, *21*, 3. [CrossRef] [PubMed]

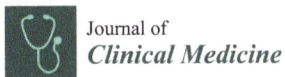

Article

Neuromonitoring of the Recurrent Laryngeal Nerve Reduces the Rate of Bilateral Vocal Cord Dysfunction in Planned Bilateral Thyroid Procedures

Constantin Smaxwil [1], Miriam Aleker [1], Julia Altmeier [1], Ali Naddaf [1], Mirjam Busch [1], Joachim Wagner [1], Simone Harsch [2], Oswald Ploner [3] and Andreas Zielke [1,*]

1. Endocrine Center Stuttgart, Department of Endocrine Surgery, Diakonie-Klinikum Stuttgart, 70176 Stuttgart, Germany; smaxwil@diak-stuttgart.de (C.S.); aleker@diak-stuttgart.de (M.A.); julia.altmeier@diak-stuttgart.de (J.A.); naddaf@diak-stuttgart.de (A.N.); buschm@diak-stuttgart.de (M.B.); wagner@diak-stuttgart.de (J.W.)
2. Outcomes Research Unit, Endocrine Center Stuttgart, Diakonie-Klinikum Stuttgart, 70176 Stuttgart, Germany; simone.harsch@diak-stuttgart.de
3. Endocrine Center Stuttgart, Department of Endocrinology, Diakonie-Klinikum Stuttgart, 70176 Stuttgart, Germany; ploner@diak-stuttgart.de
* Correspondence: ezs@diak-stuttgart.de; Tel.: +49-711-9913301; Fax: +49-711-9913309

Citation: Smaxwil, C.; Aleker, M.; Altmeier, J.; Naddaf, A.; Busch, M.; Wagner, J.; Harsch, S.; Ploner, O.; Zielke, A. Neuromonitoring of the Recurrent Laryngeal Nerve Reduces the Rate of Bilateral Vocal Cord Dysfunction in Planned Bilateral Thyroid Procedures. *J. Clin. Med.* **2021**, *10*, 740. https://doi.org/10.3390/jcm10040740

Academic Editor: Marek Ruchala and Ewelina Szczepanek-Parulska
Received: 11 November 2020
Accepted: 31 January 2021
Published: 12 February 2021

Publisher's Note: MDPI stays neutral with regard to jurisdictional claims in published maps and institutional affiliations.

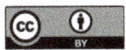

Copyright: © 2021 by the authors. Licensee MDPI, Basel, Switzerland. This article is an open access article distributed under the terms and conditions of the Creative Commons Attribution (CC BY) license (https://creativecommons.org/licenses/by/4.0/).

Abstract: Purpose: Bilateral vocal cord dysfunction (bVCD) is a rare but feared complication of thyroid surgery. This long term retrospective study determined the effect of intraoperative neuromonitoring (IONM) of the recurrent laryngeal nerve (RLN) during thyroid surgeries with regard to the rate of bVCD and evaluated the frequency as well as the outcome of staged operations. Methods: Retrospective analysis of prospectively documented data (2000–2019) of a tertiary referral centers' database. IONM started in 2000 and, since 2010, discontinuation of surgery was encouraged in planned bilateral surgeries to prevent bVCD, if non-transient loss of signal (ntLOS) occurred on the first side. Datasets of the most recent 40-month-period were assessed in detail to determine the clinical outcome of unilateral ntLOS in planned bilateral thyroid procedures. Results: Of 22,573 patients, 65 had bVCD (0.288%). The rate of bVCD decreased from 0.44 prior to 2010 to 0.09% after 2010 ($p < 0.001$, Chi2). Case reviews of the most recent 40 months period identified ntLOS in 113/3115 patients (3.6%, 2.2% NAR), of which 40 ntLOS were recorded during a planned bilateral procedure ($n = 952$, 2.1% NAR). Of 21 ntLOS occurring on the first side of the bilateral procedure, 15 procedures were stopped, subtotal contralateral resections were performed, and thyroidectomy was continued in 3 patients respectively, with the use of continuous vagal IONM. Eighteen cases of VCD were documented postop, and all but one patient had a full recovery. Seven patients had staged resections after 1 to 18 months (median 4) after the first procedure. Conclusion: IONM facilitates reduced postoperative bVCD rates. IONM is, therefore, recommendable in planned bilateral procedures. The rate of non-complete bilateral surgery after intraoperative non-transient LOS was 2%.

Keywords: thyroid surgery; vocal cord dysfunction; vocal cord palsy; loss of signal; complications

1. Introduction

Intraoperative neuromonitoring (IONM) to the recurrent laryngeal nerve (RLN) is almost always employed during thyroid surgeries in Germany. First introduced in 1996, IONM was rapidly adopted in dedicated centers of thyroid surgery and has become widely accepted in the German surgical community [1,2]. To prevent postsurgical vocal cord dysfunction (VCD), dissection of the recurrent laryngeal nerve is considered gold standard [3,4]. IONM has since received a substantial body of clinical research. It was shown early on that a "loss of signal" (LOS) of the RLN detected by means of IONM carried a substantial likelihood of postoperative vocal cord paralysis [5,6]. Acknowledging its clinical utility, the German Association of Endocrine Surgeons (CAEK) published guidelines for a standardized use, intraoperative trouble shooting and interpretation of IONM as early as 2013 [7]. Owing to the growing scientific evidence, the CAEK-guideline on thyroid surgery for benign conditions encouraged the use of IONM in 2016. Moreover, it suggested that the result of IONM could be used for intraoperative decision making. Already in 2012, a paper suggested to refrain from resection of the contralateral lobe in the case of a LOS of the RLN on the first side of the planned bilateral procedure aiming to prevent bVCD [8].

Bilateral VCD (bVCD) is a rare condition, reported to occur in 0.2–1.2% of thyroid surgeries [5,9–11]. Because bVCD is likely to cause significant obstruction of the airway, urgent respiratory therapy and tracheostomy are often needed for relief of symptoms. Although bVCD often is temporary, its impact on the affected individual as well as the health economic burden are significant. Previous reports suggest IONM of the RLN to facilitate reduced rates of bVCD [12–15]. IONM does not prevent injury to the nerve once occurred, but allows us to document an electromyographic "loss of signal" which, especially if the LOS does not recover during the procedure (i.e., non-transient LOS, ntLOS) correlates to a loss of function of the vocal cord most of the time [12–15]. It has been suggested that bVCD rates should decrease if a strategy is adopted to consider discontinuation of a bilateral procedure in the event of unilateral ntLOS. Data to support such a concept are scarce [13,15]. Moreover, little is known about the incidence as well as the outcome of staged operations in the event of a halted procedure [13,15–17].

We, therefore, analyzed our Thyroid Center Database comprising of a large patient sample over a long period of time. To this end, annual rates of bVCD prior to and after implementing IONM to check the functional integrity of the NLR were produced and the clinical outcome of a change of surgical strategy because of intraoperative ntLOS in planned bilateral thyroid procedures was analyzed in detail in the most recent period.

2. Materials and Methods

2.1. Study Population

The data presented in this publication represent a single center retrospective analysis of prospectively collected data from January 2000 to December 2019 extracted from the Quality Assurance Registry. The registry has been in use since 2000, recording all thyroid procedures with and without adverse events. Annual reports were produced for internal review. In 2009, the registry was redesigned to comply with requirements of the German Association of Endocrine Surgeons (CAEK) of the German Association of Surgeons. Since 2017, the StuDoQ registry of the DGAVC has been in use. At all times, entries into the registry were done in a prospective fashion. All data computed for this publication were pseudonymized or aggregate non-individual data.

2.2. Implementation of Intraoperative Neuromonitoring of the Recurrent Laryngeal Nerve—Reflecting the Evolution of the Use of IONM in Germany

During the 19-year period, 7 endocrine staff surgeons (including 3 changes in staff) were responsible for all of the surgeries reported here, and 4 of the 7 surgeons are still active. Until 2015, with few exemptions, all of these procedures had been total thyroidectomies and bilateral dissection to visualize the recurrent laryngeal nerve was standard. IONM was introduced in 2000, however, it was only incidentally used until 2005, where a broader application was initiated. In 2009, the decision was made to always use IONM to reassure that a dissected recurrent laryngeal nerve was well preserved and functioning. Intermittent IONM comprised stimulation of the vagal and the recurrent laryngeal nerve (RLN), was mandatory and always documented at the end of resection of either thyroid lobe. For the purpose of this study, any loss of signal that did not improve intraoperatively (i.e., non-transient LOS, either global type 2 and/or segmental type 1) and that had occurred after a functioning initial result had been obtained, was considered a potential injury to the RLN. In accordance with the literature, the term "loss of signal" (LOS) was defined and used in any event with a failure of intermittent IONM to elicit contractions of the

VC-muscle. Only if LOS persisted (i.e., was not reversible) during the time of the surgical procedure, a "non transient" LOS was recorded. At all times, evolving protocols such as the International Standards Guideline in 2010 or the German Association of Endocrine Surgeons (CAEK) Guideline in 2013 were used for intraoperative trouble shooting and verification of IONM technique [2,7]. Moreover, in the case of ntLOS, dissection of the recurrent laryngeal nerve was done to ensure morphologic integrity of the nerve.

Since 2010, surgeons were urged to reconsider continuation and/or the extent of surgery in the event of non-transient (nt) LOS on the first side of a planned bilateral procedure. As mentioned above, visual identification of RLN remained the gold standard, and intermitted IONM was used with either needle electrodes or EMG-tube electrodes (as soon as these electrodes became available). All patients had pre- and postoperative VC-tests by direct laryngoscopy on the first postoperative day by an ENT consultant of the ENT-department. Patients with preexisting unilateral or bVCD of all causes were excluded. In this institution, continuous IONM is used in selected cases, such as re-operative surgery and extensive surgery for malignant tumors of the thyroid. However, in order to compare similar endpoints at all times, only non-transient LOS were addressed in this study. To determine the effect of IONM and intraoperative decision-making, bilateral VCD rates prior to 2010 were compared to those after introduction of routine IONM and the option of staged procedures. Differences were tested for significance using Chi2 tests.

2.3. Assessing the Incidence of Procedural Change and Staged Operations

To determine the likelihood and the outcome of staged procedures, the clinical results of all thyroid surgeries during the most recent 30 months plus a 10 months follow-up period were evaluated. To this end an unselected, consecutive series of thyroid procedures including re-operative surgery as well as surgeries for malignant thyroid tumors between April 2017 to December 2019 was evaluated using the centers' StuDoQ-Database. The frequency of ntLOS during planned unilateral and bilateral thyroid procedures, voice outcome, and the frequency as well as the extent of staged procedures was determined. For this analysis, all cases with impaired motility including paresis were recorded as vocal cord dysfunction (VCD) and, therefore, include cases with a complete paresis of the vocal cord (VCP). All patients were followed per protocol with repeat laryngeal examinations by direct laryngoscopy at 6 weeks and 6 months and at 12 months if VCD persisted.

2.4. Ethics Approval and Consent to Participate

This study was approved by the Institutional Review Board of the Diakonie-Klinikum Stuttgart and conducted by the Endocrine Centers certified Outcomes Research Unit. All methods were carried out in accordance with the Declaration of Helsinki and the approved guidelines. The data enrolled in this study were obtained from the centers pseudonymized quality assurance database (since 2017 the StuDoQ-Database for certified centers of Endocrine Surgery of the German Association of Surgeons, DGAVC). Ethical committees determined that the data presented in this article do not represent a human participant research study, do not include personal identifying information, and were carried out in accordance with the relevant legislation for the purpose of quality monitoring and quality assurance. Therefore, this analysis did not require informed consent other than the consent obtained prior to entering data into the StuDoQ Database.

3. Results

3.1. The Incidence of Bilateral Vocal Cord Dysfunction in a High Volume Thyroid Center

From January 2000 until December 2017, a total of 22,573 patients with intact bilateral VC-function underwent first time surgery for benign thyroid conditions. The number of thyroid procedures per year ranged from 892–1438, with an average of some 1200 procedures p.a. IONM had been introduced in 2000, but initially was only used in selected cases. Following a decision to further the application of IONM, its use steadily increased to

50% in 2009. Since 2010, routine use of IONM had been implemented, and IONM applied in basically every patient with a thyroid procedure (Figure 1).

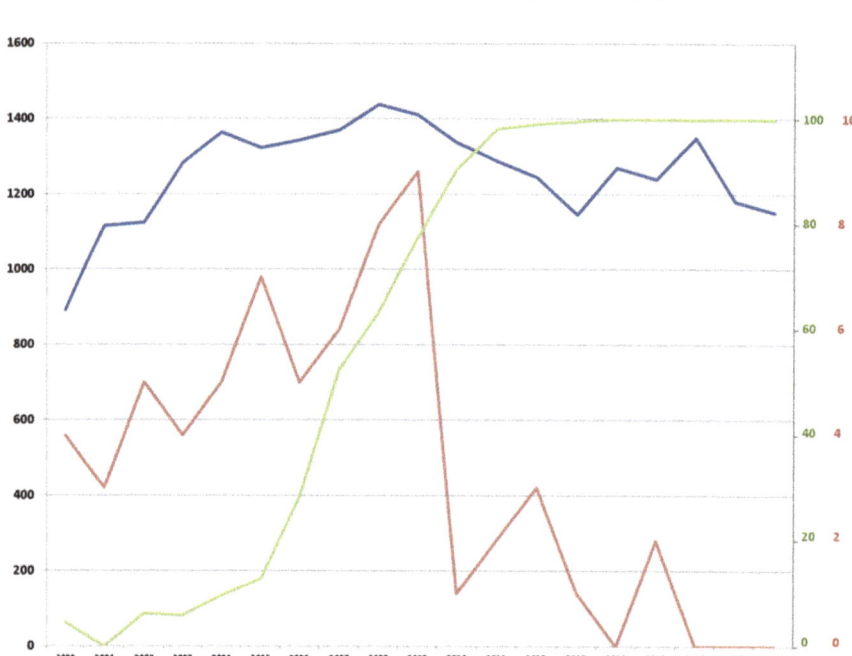

Figure 1. Synopsis of the number of thyroid procedures (scale on the left in black), percentage of procedures with intraoperative neuromonitoring (IONM) (scale on the right in green) and bilateral vocal cord dysfunction (VCD) (scale on the right in red).

During the entire period, the registry recorded a total of 65 patients to have had postoperative bVCD, for an overall rate of 0.29% (range 0–0.64% per year). The rate of bVCD prior to 2010 averaged 0.44% with a minimum of 0.27% and a maximum of 0.64% per year. With the event of routine IONM (2010–2017) and the option of staged procedures, the average rate of bVCD was recorded to be 0.09% (range 0–0.24% per year). Thus, the average rate of bVCD decreased from 0.44% to 0.09% following introduction of IONM and the option to reconsider the extent of surgery in case of a non-transient LOS (n = 56 of 12,664 vs. n = 9 of 9909 thyroid procedures, respectively; p < 0.001, Chi2). Of all patients with IONM, only one patient with bVCD had no record of any type of LOS at all (<0.01%). From 2017 onwards, there was no case of bVCD on record.

3.2. Change of Surgical Procedure in Face of a Potential Impairment of Vocal Cord Function

If an algorithm that takes account of IONM should become surgical practice, patients would need to be informed about the likelihood and the outcome of staged thyroid procedures. We detailed these events in an unselected, consecutive series. From April 2017 to December 2019 (plus a 10 months follow-up period) case reviews were obtained from the centers' StuDoQ database and comprised of all thyroid procedures, including operations for thyroid cancer (14.9%), recurrent neck surgery (8.2%), and Graves' disease (7.1%). During 3115 thyroid procedures, non-transient LOS was recorded in 113 cases (3.6%) with a rate of 2.2% per nerve at risk (NAR). Of 113 ntLOS, 100 had a documented VCD on the first postoperative day (83.3%) with a majority of cases (n = 89; 74.2%) displaying a complete paralysis of the ipsilateral vocal cord. The rate of any kind of VCD in all patients was 153/3115 (3.0% NAR), and the rate of VCD that had not completely recovered after 12 months was 22/3115. These included individuals that had either persisting VCP ($n = 7$) or were lost to follow up ($n = 15$, last observation carried on forward, LOCF). This produced a rate of persisting VCD of a minimum 0.1% and a maximum 0.4% NAR. There was no case of bVCD (Table 1).

Table 1. Synopsis of the indication for surgery, results of the pre- and postop VC assessment, and detailed numbers regarding ntLOS and VCD (April 2017–December 2019, plus 10 months follow up). VCD includes any type of impaired vocal cord function and includes vocal cord paresis (VCP).

	All Cases with IONM	3115	100%
	Multinodular Goiter	2173	69.8%
	Graves' disease	222	7.1%
	Repeat Surgery	256	8.2%
	Thyroid Cancer	464	14.9%
	Planned unilateral surgery	2163	69.4%
	Planned bilateral surgery	952	30.9%
	"Nerves at risk", NAR	5150	
VCD			
	Preoperative VC-dysfunction (VCD)	36	1.2%
	Preoperative VC-paresis (VCP)	27	0.9%
	Unilateral postop VCD	153	3.0% *
	Unilateral postop VCP	120	2.3% *
	Bilateral postop VCD	0	
ntLOS			
	VCD without nt LOS	53/153	34.6%
	VCP without nt LOS	31/120	25.8%
	Cases with nt LOS	113	
	ntLOS without VCD	20	17.7%
	ntLOS with VCD	100	83.3%
	ntLOS with VCP	89	74.2%
	Persisting VCD, min.	7	0.1% **
	Persisting VCD, max. (15 LOCF)	22	0.4% **

* % NAR; ** % NAR, data presented as a minimum rate and a hypothetical maximum rate including patients either unwilling to take a VC-test or lost to follow up and in whom the last observation of VCD is carried on forward (LOCF).

Of the 113 cases with ntLOS, 73 had been recorded during a unilateral procedure. The rate of planned bilateral operations was 952 (30.5%), and the remaining 40 cases of ntLOS were recorded within this group for an overall rate of 4.2%. Of these, 21 occurred on the first side of the procedure. A change of surgical strategy was documented in all of these cases. Procedures were halted in 15 cases, and resection of the contralateral thyroid lobe was not done. In 3 cases, the procedure was continued but restricted to a "limited" sub-total resection leaving a remnant thyroid volume at the ligament of Berry on the contralateral side—as a means to protect exposition of the most vulnerable part of the nerve. In another 3 cases, all of which were thyroid cancer, the contralateral lobe was dissected, making use of continuous vagal IONM (Figure 2).

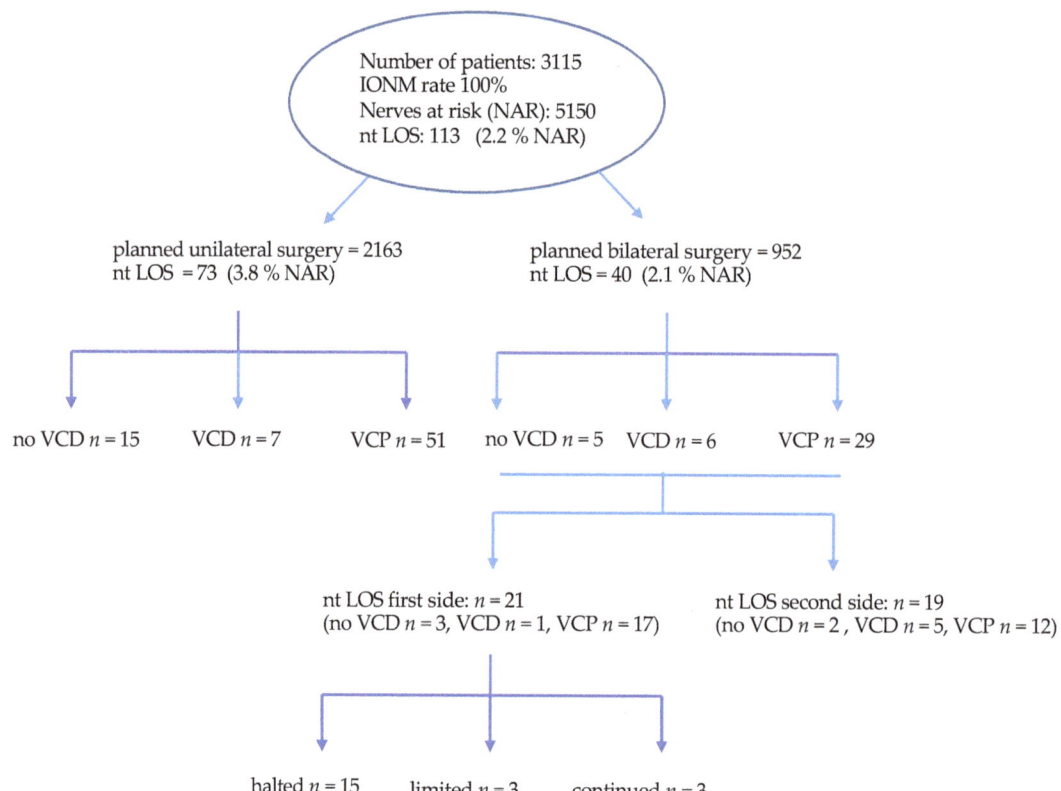

Figure 2. Flow chart depicting number of cases, uni- and bilateral thyroid procedures, events with ntLOS and the respective voice outcome, as well as the extend of thyroid gland resection.

Thus, the rate of patients with planned bilateral resections affected by a change of operative strategy was 21 out of 952 (2.2%), and the rate of non-completed resections was 18 out of 21 (1.9%). Of the 18 patients with documented VCD, impaired motility of the VC resolved in all but one after a median of 5 months. Seven patients had the second lobe removed between 1–18 (median 4) months after the primary procedure. The majority were patients with Graves' disease and differentiated thyroid cancer awaiting radioiodine ablation. Patients with multinodular goiter were less likely to have a second procedure (Table 2).

Table 2. Perioperative findings of patients with ntLOS on the 1st side of a planned bilateral procedure: Intraoperative response to LOS (continuation, limited resection, or stopping the procedure), as well as postoperative status of VC function and further treatment.

Preoperative Diagnosis	Response to Nt LOS	VCP (Months)	Further Treatment
Graves' disease	Stopped procedure	6	No completion, continued follow-up, normal TSH without medication, no sign of Endocrine Orbitopathy, full relief from preoperative symptoms
Bilat. MNG + local discomfort, recurrent goitre	Halted procedure	4	No completion, full relief from symptoms
Bilat. MNG + local discomfort	Halted procedure	Persistent	No completion
Bilat. MNG + local discomfort	Halted procedure	4	Completion thyroidectomy after 4 months
Graves disease	Halted procedure	3	Completion thyroidectomy after 5 months

Table 2. Cont.

Preoperative Diagnosis	Response to Nt LOS	VCP (Months)	Further Treatment
Bilat. MNG + local discomfort and suspicious nodule	Halted procedure	No VCD	No completion, benign histology, patient reports full relief from preoperative symptoms
Bilat. MNG + local discomfort and suspicious nodule	Halted procedure	4	No completion, benign histology, patient reports full relief from preoperative symptoms
Bilat. MNG, hyperfunctioning adenoma	Halted procedure	6	No completion, normal TSH without medication, patient reports full relief from symptoms
PTC 35 mm, pN0 (0/12)	Continued with cIONM	n.d.	Patient refuses to see ENT specialist, claims full control of voice during follow up visits
Bilat. MNG with local discomfort + primary hyperparathyroidism	Continued with cIONM **	12	** Dunhill procedure, leaving contralateral upper pole, procedure continued because of contralateral parathyroid adenoma and hypercalcaemia
Bilat. MNG + local discomfort	Continued with cIONM **	no VCD	** "Limited" resection of a contralateral nodule close to the isthmus, remnant lobe size: 3 mL
Bilat. MNG + local discomfort	Halted procedure	6	No completion, patient reports full relief from preoperative symptoms
Bilat. MNG + bilat. autonomus nodules	Halted procedure	6	Completion thyroidectomy after 9 months
PTC at multiple sites, 7 mm, pN0 (0/5)	Continued with cIONM	4	Radioiodine treatment
Graves disease	Halted procedure	4	Completion rejected, radioiodine for persisting Graves' after 8 months
Bilat. MNG + local discomfort and Hashimoto	Halted procedure	3	No completion, patient reports full relief from preoperative symptoms
PTC 8 mm, pN1 (11/37)	Halted procedure	1	Completion thyroidectomy and completion LAD after 2 months, radioiodine therapy
Graves disease	Halted procedure	3	Completion thyroidectomy after 4 months
PTC 18 mm, pN1 (3/8)	Continued with cIONM	3	Radioiodine treatment
Bilat. MNG + local discomfort	Continued with cIONM **	4	** "Limited" contralateral, subtotal resection leaving a remnant of 5 mL
PTC 25 mm, pN (0/16)	Continued with IONM **	no VCD	** Procedure continued after temporary LOS on 1st side, contralateral resection and LAD; nt-LOS of the 1st side (type II) documented at final assessment
Graves disease	Halted procedure	1	Completion thyroidectomy after 2 months

4. Discussion

In 2017, some 70,000 patients underwent surgery of the thyroid gland in Germany [18]. Almost two thirds of these operations addressed both thyroid lobes, and the majority were total thyroidectomies [11]. Recurrent laryngeal nerve (RLN) injury is a feared complication and prevention of postsurgical vocal cord dysfunction (VCD) during thyroid surgery is paramount. However, the true rate of postsurgical unilateral VCD is not precisely known. Based on data from prospective trials, the risk of permanent VCD has been estimated to be around 3% in expert centers [5,6,8]. Health maintenance organizations in Germany estimated the rate of unilateral permanent VCD to be at least 1.5% [16]. A recent prospective analysis in a larger sample found a rate of 10.6% transient and 1.1% permanent VCD, respectively [11].

Although unilateral VCD can already be a significant limitation and occasionally may lead to incapacity to work, bilateral VCD can be much more demanding including the need for tracheostomy [17,19]. Friedrich et al. reported a rate of a permanent bilateral VCD of 0.3% and found the immediate postoperative symptoms of bilateral VCD to be variable—

from the rare patient with very little symptoms to severely impaired patients suffering from dysphonia, dyspnea, and extreme stridor [20]. In such cases, temporary ventilation support and permanent tracheotomy are necessary [19]. With respect to the likelihood of VCD, previous research has determined the surgeon to be the most important risk factor. There is cumulative evidence to support the concept, that the individual risk decreases with the number of surgeries per surgeon. Moreover, malignant disease and secondary surgery are additional risk factors [5,16]. Even with careful dissection of the RLN and experience, unilateral and rarely bilateral VCD may also occur.

With the advent of IONM, hopes were raised that IONM would prevent injury to the nerve, but this has yet to be shown. Whether or not continuous IONM does have the potential to facilitate reduced VCD rates has yet to be established [6,11]. However, permanent loss of neurophysiological nerve signal (LOS) during surgery is highly indicative of an injury to the nerve [12–15]. This study confirmed that two thirds of patients with nt LOS have postoperative VCD (Table 1). Therefore, IONM may have the potential to assist surgeons, reassuring the functional integrity of the nerve to have been preserved, which is especially important in bilateral thyroid surgeries. The relevance is underscored by the 2.2% rate of ntLOS on the first side of bilateral procedures found in this study. The data of this study show the number of bilateral events to decrease with the use of IONM: From 1 in 200 to less than 1 in a 1000 procedures. On the other hand, and in order to reduce the number of patients affected by bilateral VCD, changes in surgical strategy including incomplete and halted resections are necessary. This concept was first published in 2012 [8,13]. Patients would need to be informed about the likelihood and the outcome of a staged procedure, but until now only a small number of studies have reported on surgical outcomes [8,14,21]. We have found the likelihood of a change of surgical strategy to be around 3% and the rate of incomplete resections to be around 2% in planned bilateral surgeries comparing well to previous reports [14,21].

Moreover, a halted procedure in patients with benign nodular thyroid disease allows for a critical appraisal of clinical signs and symptoms after removal of the dominant thyroid lobe—and may not always require a complete thyroidectomy. This contrasts a recent suggestion to start a bilateral procedure on the side of the smaller of the two thyroid lobes—in order to get more space to safely dissect the larger one [22]. We aim to start the procedure on the side of the dominant lobe allowing us to entertain the option of a halted procedure after removal of the most significant lobe. It is, however, noteworthy that the likelihood to halt the procedure or to continue surgery differs between countries. In Germany, most endocrine and thyroid surgeons would be willing to discontinue surgery in case of ntLOS [8], whereas in France, most of the surgeons would continue [23]. It would, however, be reasonable to assume that along with the increasing use of IONM, an increasing acceptance to refrain from bilateral surgery in the event of unilateral ntLOS may be seen [24,25]. Recently, authors from the UK recommend staged thyroidectomies only for "less experienced surgeons" [22]. Although, one should be reminded, however small an experienced surgeons' rate of postoperative VCD may be, continuing surgery after ntLOS on the first side will always carry a discernable risk of bVCD with the potential of life-threatening consequences.

There are some limitations of this study for critical discussion. This is not a stringent prospective observational trial. It is a report of real-world data from a thyroid surgery registry over a rather large period of time. As such, it reflects the technical evolution of the application and interpretation of IONM. However, as outlined in this report, bVCD is quite rare and prospective studies, until now, have failed to bring forward numbers large enough to sufficiently address the use of IONM in this rare event. Moreover, valid data from prospective multi-institutional registries are currently not available, but may be published in forthcoming years [11].

Another weakness of this study is that the registry only allowed for a correlation of non-transitory LOS with postoperative VCD. Transient LOS or "combined events" were recorded only after 2015 and 2017, respectively. When IONM was introduced and until

2010, these events had yet to be named and to be properly characterized. However, ntLOS is a clear cut and decided endpoint of IONM, that requires no interpretation and, as such, can readily be used for intraoperative decision making. This study has confirmed, as others have, that ntLOS carries a rather high likelihood of postoperative VDP. Nevertheless, the considerable rate of VCD without ntLOS documented in this study indicates the future potential of continuous IONM. Whenever intermittent IONM is used, there is a possibility of missed transient events of impaired signaling which might be a sign of nerve damage. In fact, early experience with continuous IONM indicates that impaired transduction of signal may be used to alter the surgical approach to the NLR and avoid injury. However, this observation awaits confirmation by a PRCCT [6].

Finally, this study did not evaluate the relationship between LOS, the extent of a bilateral surgical procedure, the weight of the specimen removed or the results of histopathology. It only addressed the event of unilateral or bilateral VCD. However, from a patient's perspective this may be the most relevant factor.

Despite these limitations, this large single institution database from a rather small number of responsible surgeons could minimize the possibility of inconsistency of clinical data, surgical technique, and intraoperative management policy. We are, therefore, quite confident, that our finding of IONM to be a useful application in bilateral thyroid procedures is to be reassured during more elaborate future trials.

In conclusion, we believe this study demonstrated that intraoperative non-transitory LOS mandates reconsideration of the thyroid procedure and that this may change the overall surgical outcome to the better. Postoperative bVCD rates can be reduced by means of IONM and taking account of intraoperative ntLOS. We believe that IONM should be available in every case of a planned bilateral thyroid procedure. We found the likelihood of an incomplete surgical procedure as a result of such intraoperative decision-making to be around 2%.

Author Contributions: Conceptualization, C.S., O.P., and A.Z.; methodology, C.S., A.Z.; software, S.H.; validation, C.S., S.H. and A.Z.; investigation, J.W.; resources, M.B.; data curation, M.A., A.N., J.A., and C.S.; writing—original draft preparation, C.S., A.Z.; final review and editing, C.S., O.P., and A.Z.; visualization, S.H. All authors have read and agreed to the published version of the manuscript.

Funding: Authors state no funding involved.

Data Availability Statement: Restrictions apply to the data presented in this study. Data were obtained from the StuDoQ Thyroid Quality Assurance Registry of the German Association of Surgeons (DGAVC) and may be available to third parties only upon request to the SAVC/DGAVC and decision at the discretion of the DGAVC.

Conflicts of Interest: The authors declare no competing interests.

Abbreviations

bVCD	bilateral vocal cord dysfunction
IONM	intraoperative neuromonitoring
cIONM	continuous intraoperative neuromonitoring
LOCF	last observation carried forward
LOS	loss of signal; ntLOS, non transient LOS
NAR	nerves at risk
RLNP	paresis of the recurrent laryngeal nerve
StuDoQ	Thyroid surgery registry of the German Association of Surgeons; StuDoQ I Thyroid
VC	vocal cord
VCD	vocal cord dysfunction
VCP	vocal cord paresis

References

1. Eisele, D.W. Intraoperative Electrophysiologic Monitoring of the Recurrent Laryngeal Nerve. *Laryngoscope* **1996**, *106*, 443–449. [CrossRef] [PubMed]

2. Dionigi, G.; Chiang, F.Y.; Rausei, S.; Wu, C.W.; Boni, L.; Lee, K.W.; Rovera, F.; Cantone, G.; Bacuzzi, A. Surgical anatomy and neurophysiology of the vagus nerve (VN) for standardized intraoperative neuromonitoring (IONM) of the inferior laryngeal nerve (ILN) during thyroidectomy. *Langenbeck's Arch. Surg.* **2010**, *395*, 893–898. [CrossRef]
3. Schilling, M.K.; Seiler, C.; Schäfer, M.; Büchler, M.W. Prevention of N. recurrens paresis after thyroidectomy—A meta-analysis. *Ther. Umsch. Rev. Ther.* **1999**, *56*, 396–399. [CrossRef]
4. Dionigi, G.; Wu, C.-W.; Lombardi, D.; Accorona, R.; Bozzola, A.; Kim, H.Y.; Chiang, F.-Y.; Bignami, M.; Castelnuovo, P.; Nicolai, P. The Current State of Recurrent Laryngeal Nerve Monitoring for Thyroid Surgery. *Curr. Otorhinolaryngol. Rep.* **2013**, *2*, 44–54. [CrossRef]
5. Dralle, H.; Sekulla, C.; Haerting, J.; Timmermann, W.; Neumann, H.J.; Kruse, E.; Grond, S.; Mühlig, H.P.; Richter, C.; Voss, J.; et al. Risk factors of paralysis and functional outcome after recurrent laryngeal nerve monitoring in thyroid surgery. *Surgery* **2004**, *136*, 1310–1322. [CrossRef]
6. Schneider, R.; Machens, A.; Randolph, G.W.; Kamani, D.; Lorenz, K.; Dralle, H. Opportunities and challenges of intermittent and continuous intraoperative neural monitoring in thyroid surgery. *Gland. Surg.* **2017**, *6*, 537–545. [CrossRef] [PubMed]
7. Randolph, G.W.; Dralle, H. Electrophysiologic recurrent laryngeal nerve monitoring during thyroid and parathyroid surgery: International standards guideline statement. *Laryngoscope* **2011**, *121* (Suppl. 1), 1–16. [CrossRef] [PubMed]
8. Dralle, H.; Sekulla, C.; Lorenz, K.; Thanh, P.N.; Schneider, R.; Machens, A. Loss of the nerve monitoring signal during bilateral thyroid surgery. *BJS* **2012**, *99*, 1089–1095. [CrossRef] [PubMed]
9. Thomusch, O.; Dralle, H. *Schilddrüsenchirurgie: Kostenanalyse und Qualitätssicherung*; Barth: Heidelberg, Germany, 1997.
10. Affleck, B.D.; Swartz, K.; Brennan, J. Surgical considerations and controversies in thyroid and parathyroid surgery. *Otolaryngol. Clin. North Am.* **2003**, *36*, 159–187. [CrossRef]
11. Bartsch, D.K.; Dotzenrath, C.; Vorländer, C.; Zielke, A.; Weber, T.; Buhr, H.J.; Klinger, C.; Lorenz, K.; StuDoQ/Thyroid Study Group. Current practice of surgery for benign goiter—An analysis of the prospective German Association of Surgeons DGAV StuDoQ|Thyroid Registry. *J. Clin. Med.* **2019**, *8*, 477. [CrossRef] [PubMed]
12. Calò, P.G.; Medas, F.; Erdas, E.; Pittau, M.R.; Demontis, R.; Pisano, G.; Nicolosi, A. Role of intraoperative neuromonitoring of recurrent laryngeal nerves in the outcomes of surgery for thyroid cancer. *Int. J. Surg.* **2014**, *12*, S213–S217. [CrossRef]
13. Melin, M.; Schwarz, K.; Lammers, B.J.; Goretzki, P.E. IONM-guided goiter surgery leading to two-stage thyroidectomy—Indication and results. *Langenbeck's Arch. Surg.* **2013**, *398*, 411–418. [CrossRef] [PubMed]
14. Sitges-Serra, A.; Fontané, J.; Dueñas, J.P.; Duque, C.S.; Lorente, L.; Trillo, L.; Sancho, J.J. Prospective study on loss of signal on the first side during neuromonitoring of the recurrent laryngeal nerve in total thyroidectomy. *BJS* **2013**, *100*, 662–666. [CrossRef] [PubMed]
15. Schneider, R.; Lorenz, K.; Sekulla, C.; Machens, A.; Nguyen-Thanh, P.; Dralle, H. Surgical strategy during intended total thyroidectomy after loss of EMG signal on the first side of resection. *Chirurg* **2015**, *86*, 154–163. [CrossRef] [PubMed]
16. Wissenschaftliches Instituts der AOK (WIdO). *Final Report: QSR: Entwicklung des Leistungsbereichs Operation bei Benigner Schilddrüsenerkrankung*; Oktober: Berlin, Germany, 2015; p. 39.
17. Calò, P.G.; Medas, F.; Conzo, G.; Podda, F.; Canu, G.L.; Gambardella, C.; Pisano, G.; Erdas, E.; Nicolosi, A. Intraoperative neuromonitoring in thyroid surgery: Is the two-staged thyroidectomy justified? *Int. J. Surg.* **2017**, *41*, S13–S20. [CrossRef] [PubMed]
18. Statistisches Bundesamt DESTATIS. *Fallpauschalenbezogene Fallstatistik: DRG Statistik. Operationen und Prozeduren der Vollstationären Patientinnen und Patienten in Krankenhäusern*; Statistisches Bundesam: Berlin, Germany, 2017.
19. Joliat, G.R.; Guarnero, V.; Demartines, N.; Schweizer, V.; Matter, M. Recurrent laryngeal nerve injury after thyroid and parathyroid surgery: Incidence and postoperative evolution assessment. *Medicine* **2017**, *96*, e6674. [CrossRef]
20. Friedrich, T.; Eichfeld, U.; Hänsch, U.; Dähnert, I.; Steinert, M.; Schönfelder, M. Häufigkeit und klinische Symptomatik der doppelseitigen Recurrensparese nach Schilddrüsenoperation. In *Vielfalt und Einheit der Chirurgie Humanität und Wissenschaft*; Hartel, W., Ed.; Langenbecks Archiv für Chirurgie: Berlin, Germany, 1998.
21. Schneider, R.; Randolph, G.W.; Sekulla, C.; Phelan, E.; Thanh, P.N.; Bucher, M.; Machens, A.; Dralle, H.; Lorenz, K. Continuous intraoperative vagal nerve stimulation for identification of imminent recurrent laryngeal nerve injury. *Head Neck* **2013**, *35*, 1591–1598. [CrossRef]
22. Sitges-Serra, A.; Gallego-Otaegui, L.; Fontané, J.; Trillo, L.; Lorente-Poch, L.; Sancho, J. Contralateral surgery in patients scheduled for total thyroidectomy with initial loss or absence of signal during neural monitoring. *BJS* **2019**, *106*, 404–411. [CrossRef]
23. Khamsy, L.; Constanthin, P.E.; Sadowski, S.M.; Triponez, F. Loss of neuromonitoring signal during bilateral thyroidectomy: No systematic change in operative strategy according to a survey of the French Association of Endocrine Surgeons (AFCE). *BMC Surg.* **2015**, *15*, 95. [CrossRef]
24. Sadowski, S.M.; Soardo, P.B.; Leuchter, I.; Robert, J.H.; Triponez, F. Systematic Use of Recurrent Laryngeal Nerve Neuromonitoring Changes the Operative Strategy in Planned Bilateral Thyroidectomy. *Thyroid* **2013**, *23*, 329–333. [CrossRef]
25. Schneider, R.; Randolph, G.W.; Dionigi, G.; Wu, C.W.; Barczynski, M.; Chiang, F.Y.; Al-Quaryshi, Z.; Angelos, P.; Brauckhoff, K.; Cernea, C.R.; et al. International neural monitoring study group guideline 2018 part I: Staging bilateral thyroid surgery with monitoring loss of signal. *Laryngoscope* **2018**, *128* (Suppl. 3), 1–17.

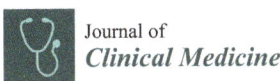

Journal of
Clinical Medicine

Article

Application of Tissue Aspirate Parathyroid Hormone Assay for Imaging Suspicious Neck Lesions in Patients with Complicated Recurrent or Persistent Renal Hyperparathyroidism

Chien-Ling Hung [1,2], Yu-Chen Hsu [3], Shih-Ming Huang [2,4] and Chung-Jye Hung [2,*]

1 Department of Surgery, Tainan Sin Lau Hospital, Tainan 704302, Taiwan; olen1981@gmail.com
2 Division of General Surgery, Department of Surgery, National Cheng Kung University Hospital, College of Medicine, National Cheng Kung University, Tainan 704302, Taiwan; smhuang@mail.ncku.edu.tw
3 Department of Surgery, Chia-Yi Christian Hospital, Chia-Yi 600566, Taiwan; seetowhat@yahoo.com.tw
4 Asian International Thyroid Center, Chang Bing Show Chwan Memorial Hospital, Changhua 505029, Taiwan
* Correspondence: cjhung@mail.ncku.edu.tw; Tel.: +886-6-2353535 (ext. 5232)

Abstract: Background: Comprehensive pre-reoperative localization is essential in complicated persistent or recurrent renal hyperparathyroidism. The widely used imaging studies sometimes lead to ambiguous results. Our study aimed to clarify the role of tissue aspirate parathyroid hormone (PTH) assay with a new positive assay definition for imaging suspicious neck lesions in these challenging scenarios. Methods: All patients with complicated recurrent or persistent renal hyperparathyroidism underwent parathyroid sonography and scintigraphy. Echo-guided tissue aspirate PTH assay was performed in suspicious lesions revealed by localization imaging studies. The tissue aspirate PTH level was determined by an immunoradiometric assay. We proposed a newly-developed definition for positive assay as a washout level higher than one-thirtieth of the serum PTH level obtained at the same time. The final diagnosis after re-operation was confirmed by the pathologists. Results: In total, 50 tissue aspirate PTH assays were performed in 32 patients with imaging suspicious neck lesions, including discrepant results between scintigraphy and sonography in 47 lesions (94%), unusual locations in 19 lesions (38%), multiple foci in 28 lesions (56%), and locations over previously explored areas in 31 lesions (62%). Among 39 assay-positive lesions, 13 lesions (33.3%) were not identified by parathyroid scintigraphy, and 28 lesions (71.8%) had uncertain parathyroid sonography findings. The final pathology in patients who underwent re-operative surgery proved the tissue aspirate PTH assays had a 100% positive predictive value. Conclusions: Our findings suggest tissue aspirate PTH assay with this new positive assay definition is beneficial to clarify the nature of imaging suspicious lesions in patients with complicated persistent or recurrent renal hyperparathyroidism.

Keywords: tissue aspirate parathyroid hormone assay; recurrent renal hyperparathyroidism; persistent renal hyperparathyroidism; parathyroid sonography; parathyroid scintigraphy

1. Introduction

Renal hyperparathyroidism is a common complication of chronic kidney disease and renal failure that can be further classified into secondary hyperparathyroidism or tertiary hyperparathyroidism according to the serum calcium level and the underlying mechanism of elevated parathyroid hormone (PTH) [1]. Improving medical treatment with vitamin D analogs, phosphate binders, and calcimimetic drugs expands the treatment options for these patients, but surgical treatment with parathyroidectomy remains necessary for many patients. The management of persistent or recurrent renal hyperparathyroidism is especially challenging for endocrine surgeons. Around 2.7–11.5% of patients needed reoperation due to persistence or recurrence after the primary operation [2–4]. However, such procedures are difficult and have a high complication rate due to adhesion, dense scar tissue, distortion of anatomic tissue, and loss of the normal plane [5]. It is generally agreed

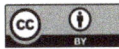

that accurate pre-reoperative localization is the cornerstone to reduce surgical risk and avoid negative neck exploration.

Parathyroid scintigraphy and sonography are the most widely used pre-reoperative localization methods. However, their sensitivity and accuracy are unsatisfactory and vary in different studies [6–9]. The accuracy of parathyroid scintigraphy is highly dependent on the size and functional status of the parathyroid glands, and thyroid lesions can lead to misinterpretations of the results [10,11]. The reported success rates of the pre-operative localization of parathyroid scintigraphy for reoperative renal hyperparathyroidism range from 71% to 93% in some small-sized studies [2,8,12], but the data remain scarce for patients with secondary or tertiary hyperparathyroidism [13]. Parathyroid sonography depends on the technical ability of the operator [14], and it is not uncommon for the findings to confuse thyroid nodules or lymph nodes. The results of parathyroid sonography for pre-reoperative localization in persistent or recurrent renal hyperparathyroidism are unsatisfactory, with a 50% sensitivity rate and a 16.7% false-positive rate shown in different studies [7,15]. Moreover, the interpretation can be complicated if there are uncertain or even discrepant results between these two localization studies. Therefore, another adjuvant tool to further clarify the results of localization studies is clearly needed.

The tissue aspirate parathyroid hormone (PTH) assay was first introduced in patients with primary hyperparathyroidism in 1983 by Doppman [16], and it is now also applied in patients with persistent or recurrent primary hyperparathyroidism featuring high sensitivity and specificity [17–19]. Nevertheless, no previous studies have reported the application of tissue aspirate PTH assays in patients with persistent or recurrent renal hyperparathyroidism. Therefore, in this study, we aimed to investigate the role of the tissue aspirate PTH assay with a new proposed positive assay definition for suspicious neck lesions for imaging in patients with complicated recurrent or persistent renal hyperparathyroidism.

2. Materials and Methods

2.1. Study Population

Patients with recurrent or persistent renal hyperparathyroidism who underwent localization studies between September 1995 and December 2014 at National Cheng Kung University Hospital (NCKUH) were enrolled in the study. Persistent renal hyperparathyroidism was defined as a PTH level higher than the upper normal range after the first operation [3]. Recurrent renal hyperparathyroidism was defined by a PTH level that dropped to or below a normal range after the first operation and rose above the normal range after 6 months [3]. All patients underwent localization studies including parathyroid sonography (neck and graft site) and parathyroid scintigraphy (neck, mediastinum, and graft site). An echo-guided tissue aspirate PTH assay was performed in each patient with suspicious or discrepant lesions revealed by the imaging results, either through sonography or scintigraphy. Informed consent was obtained from each patient before the procedure. The study was approved by the Institutional Ethics Review Board of NCKUH (A-ER-108-167).

2.2. Tissue Aspirate PTH Assay

Echo-guided tissue aspiration was performed by a single surgeon (C.J.H). The patients were asked to lie on a bed with their necks extended. After sterile preparation, the operator performed tissue aspiration with the dominant hand and held the sonography probe for localization with the other hand. A 23-gauge needle was inserted into the suspicious neck lesion under ultrasound guidance. After insertion, the operator fixed the needle and rapidly oscillated the piston 5~8 times. The aspirate was then washed out with 6 mL normal saline and sent for PTH measurement, using an immunoradiometric assay for intact PTH (Cisbio Bioassays, Codolet, France. normal range of 10–65 pg/mL), which was then compared with the serum PTH level measured before the procedure. The positive result was defined as a tissue aspirate PTH level higher than one-thirtieth of the serum

PTH level. The patients were able to leave the clinic after compression of the aspiration site for 30 min. Parathyroidectomy was suggested in assay-positive cases.

2.3. Data Analysis

The patients received follow-ups until the end of June 2017. All data on demographics, localization, tissue aspirate PTH assay results, reoperative findings and procedures, pathological findings, and post-reoperative course were recorded and analyzed. The results of parathyroid sonography were classified as either suspicious or positive, and the results of parathyroid scintigraphy were classified as negative, suspicious, or positive. The suspicious parathyroid sonographic results were defined as neck lesions with unusual locations or atypical sonographic images including shape, size, and number (Figure 1). The results of parathyroid scintigraphy were determined with the agreement of both the surgeon and nuclear medicine specialist. The final diagnosis after reoperation was confirmed by the pathologists. The accuracy of the tissue aspirate PTH assays was calculated according to the reoperative results.

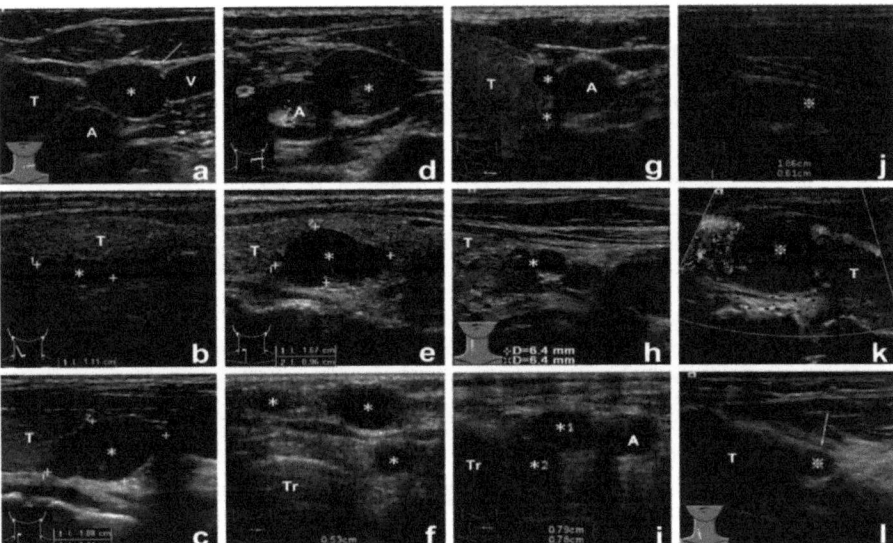

Figure 1. Images of positive and suspicious parathyroid sonography lesions. (**a**–**c**) Case 1, 2, 6, with positive sonographic lesions. (**d**) Case 5, with suspicious left upper neck lesion. (**e**) Case 20, with suspicious intrathyroid lesion. (**f**) Case 24, with suspicious multiple subcutaneous lesions. (**g**) Case 25, with suspicious dumbbell shape lesion. (**h**) Case 8, with suspicious infrathyroid lobulated lesion. (**i**) Case 26-1, with suspicious multiple paratracheal lesions. (**j**) Case 14, with suspicious intrathymus lesion (false assay-negative). (**k**) Case 31, with suspicious intrathyroid lesion. (**l**) Case 26-2, with suspicious infrathyroid small lesion. ✱ Positive tissue aspirate PTH assay lesions. ✲ Negative tissue aspirate PTH assay lesions. Demographic data of enrolled patients are listed in Table S1. Abbreviations: A, common carotid artery; V, internal jugular vein; T, thyroid; Tr, trachea.

2.4. Statistical Analysis

Continuous variables are expressed as the median and range unless stated otherwise. Categorical variables were expressed as numbers and percentages. Statistical significance was assessed by a Mann–Whitney U-test for continuous variables, and by a chi-square test and Fisher's exact test for categorical variables. All analyses were performed using the SPSS software (SPSS Statistics for Windows, Version 17.0, SPSS Inc., Chicago, IL, USA). A p value < 0.05 was considered to be statistically significant.

3. Results

3.1. Patient Demographics

In total, 115 patients with recurrent or persistent renal hyperparathyroidism underwent localization studies during the study period, and 50 tissue aspirate PTH assays were performed in 32 patients. The demographic data of the patients receiving tissue aspirate PTH assays are shown in Table S1. The mean age of these patients was 56.6 ± 7.6 years with female predominance (78.1%). Nine (28.1%) patients received their initial operation at another hospital, and eight patients (25%) underwent more than one operation before the tissue aspirate PTH assay. Four or more parathyroid glands were removed during a previous surgery in at least 21 patients (65.6%). Twenty-four patients were classified as having persistent renal hyperparathyroidism and eight as having recurrent renal hyperparathyroidism. The indications for tissue aspiration in these 50 lesions were: uncertain or discrepant results between parathyroid scintigraphy and sonography in 47 lesions (94%), unusual locations in 19 lesions (38%), multiple foci in 28 lesions (56%), and locations over previously explored areas in 31 lesions (62%). Eleven patients received two or more tissue aspirate PTH assays for multiple suspicious neck lesions at the same time, and two patients received several tissue aspirate PTH assays at different times. The median serum systemic PTH level before aspiration was 744.25 pg/mL (range 214.78 to >2500.00 pg/mL). Thirty-nine tissue aspirate PTH assays (78%) were positive. After the procedure, no complications were noted after the procedure, such as hemorrhaging, infections, persistent pain, or parathyromatosis.

3.2. Comparison between Different Assay Results

The results of the comparison between positive and negative tissue aspirate PTH assays are shown in Table 1. The median tissue aspirate PTH level was 3.9 pg/mL in the assay-negative group and 2500 pg/mL in the assay-positive group ($p < 0.001$). In contrast, there was no significant difference in the levels of serum systemic PTH and calcium between the two groups. A significant correlation was identified between the results of the parathyroid scintigraphy and tissue aspirate PTH assays ($p = 0.008$), whereas no significant correlation was found between the results of parathyroid sonography and tissue aspirate PTH assays ($p = 0.114$).

Table 1. Comparison between cohorts with positive and negative tissue aspirate PTH assays.

Tissue Aspirate PTH Assay	Negative	Positive	p Value
Number (n = 50)	11	39	
Tissue aspirate PTH level (pg/mL), median (range)	3.9 (1.0–28.6)	2500 (38.9–44470.0)	<0.001
Serum systemic PTH level (pg/mL), median (range)	428.2 (214.8–1817.8)	869.7 (227.8 ≥ 2500.0)	0.137
Serum calcium level (mg/dL), median (range)	10.0 (9.4–12.5)	10.5 (8.8–12.5)	0.218
Parathyroid scintigraphy, n (%)			0.008
Negative	9 (81.8%)	13 (33.3%)	
Suspicious	0 (0.0%)	18 (46.2%)	
Positive	2 (18.2%)	8 (20.5%)	
Parathyroid sonography, n (%)			0.114
Suspicious	11 (100%)	28 (71.8%)	
Positive	0 (0%)	11 (28.2%)	
Neck lesion explored, n (%)	3 (27.3%) †	35 (89.76%) ‡	<0.001
Pathology proved parathyroid lesions, n	1	35	

† In 3 assay-negative lesions, neck exploration was performed due to borderline assay result (1 pathology proved parathyroid lesion) and concomitant exploration in the same operation field with the other assay-positive lesions. ‡ In 4 assay-positive lesions, neck exploration was not performed due to presumed severe adhesion and controllable PTH levels in these patients. Abbreviation: PTH, parathyroid hormone.

3.3. Comparisons with Localization Studies

Comparisons between the results of tissue aspirate PTH assays and localization studies are shown in Table 2. Among the 50 lesions, three (6%) of them were triple-positive, indicating positive parathyroid scintigraphy, sonography results, and positive tissue aspirate PTH assays. Of the remaining 47 lesions that had uncertain or conflicting localization results between the parathyroid scintigraphy and sonography, 36 were assay-positive (72%) and 11 were assay-negative (22%).

Table 2. Correlation of the results between tissue aspirate PTH assays and localization studies.

Localization Studies		Parathyroid Sonography			
		Suspicious (n = 39)		Positive (n = 11)	
Parathyroid Scintigraphy	Tissue Aspirate PTH Assay	Negative (n = 11)	Positive (n = 28)	Negative (n = 0)	Positive (n = 11)
Negative (n = 22)	Negative (n = 9)	9		0	
	Positive (n = 13)		9		4
Suspicious (n = 18)	Negative (n = 0)	0		0	
	Positive (n = 18)		14		4
Positive (n = 10)	Negative (n = 2)	2 *		0	
	Positive (n = 8)		5		3

* One false-negative tissue aspirate PTH assay included. Abbreviation: PTH, parathyroid hormone.

3.4. Surgical Intervention

Thirty-five assay-positive (35/39, 90%) and three assay-negative lesions (3/11, 27%) in 26 patients were explored through neck incisions. All assay-positive and one assay-negative lesions (case 14) were pathologically proven to be parathyroid tissues. Explorations were performed for case 14 because of the uncertainty of the tissue aspiration procedure, which offered borderline assay results. In the other two true assay-negative lesions (case 26-1, 29), removal of the lesions was arranged due to concomitant exploration in the same operation field for other reasons. No surgery was performed for the four assay-positive lesions in the three patients because of presumed severe adhesion from previous management (4 times neck operations and 8 times alcohol injections, case 30) and controllable PTH levels (case 15, 21). The median weight of resected parathyroid glands was 878.0 mg (range 193.0 to 3674.0 mg). In the lesions for which surgery was performed, the positive predictive value of tissue aspirate PTH assays was 100%.

3.5. Reoperative Findings

The reoperative findings are shown in Table 3. Among the 36 parathyroid lesions in the 26 patients who underwent surgery, six lesions were ectopic parathyroids, nine lesions were parathyromatosis, and eight lesions were intrathyroid parathyroids. The other 13 lesions were located over the usual parathyroid areas that had already been explored during previous surgical procedures.

Table 3. Location of parathyroid lesions removed during reoperations.

Location	Lesions (n = 36)	Patients (n = 26) *
Ectopic		
Undescended	3 (8.3%)	3
Intrathymic	1 (2.8%)	1
Carotid sheath	2 (5.6%)	2
Parathyromatosis	9 (25.0%)	4
Intrathyroid	8 (22.2%)	7
Neck (usual parathyroid area)		
LS	4 (11.1%)	4
LI	1 (2.8%)	1
RS	4 (11.1%)	4
RI	4 (11.1%)	4

* Seven patients had two or more assay-positive lesions removed during the same operation. Abbreviations: LS: left superior; LI: left inferior; RS: right superior; RI: right inferior.

4. Discussion

In our series, among the patients who received reoperations, 16.7% of the lesions were ectopic, 22.2% were intrathyroid, 36.1% were located over previously explored areas, and 25.0% lesions were confirmed to be parathyromatosis in this study. In challenging medical scenarios, experienced surgeons need comprehensive pre-reoperative localization information to ensure that treatment is achieved. The elevated tissue aspirate PTH assays found with our newly proposed positive assay definitions may help surgeons identify suspicious neck lesions discovered in localization imaging studies with a high positive predictive value (100%) and effectively avoid negative neck explorations in such complicated cases.

Although tissue aspirate PTH assays can help confirm parathyroid tissue for suspicious neck lesions, not all neck lesions need this examination. We suggest this procedure be reserved for suspicious neck lesions with uncertain or discrepant localization study results, lesions with unusual locations or numbers, lesions over previously explored areas, or a combination of these findings. One of the reasons to use tissue aspirate PTH assays sparingly is the potential for seeding and causing parathyromatosis. To avoid such complications, including seeding along the needle tract, fibrotic tissue reaction, and potential reactive changes of parathyroid lesions [20], the operator should fix the needle and simply oscillate the piston with negative pressure following the needle's introduction into the center of the suspicious lesion instead of moving the needle tip back and forth, as in other studies [17,19,21].

From our series, we found that 71.8% (28/39) of the lesions with positive tissue aspirate PTH assays were considered to be uncertain (suspicious) by parathyroid sonography. Among the positive tissue aspirate PTH assays with uncertain sonographic lesions, 82% (23/28) were scintigraphy-negative or scintigraphy-suspicious lesions. Therefore, tissue aspirate PTH assays may help in identifying lesions that potentially need intervention. Moreover, without the application of tissue aspirate PTH assays, at least nine (23.1%) of the lesions with positive tissue aspirate PTH assays could have been easily missed based on the localization results (negative parathyroid scintigraphy and uncertain parathyroid sonography).

There is no established standard for the level of PTH that is considered to indicate positive evidence that the aspirated tissue represents parathyroid tissue. Theoretically, the level of PTH in nonparathyroid tissue should be undetectable, as described in a prior study [22]. There have been different positive tissue aspirate PTH values recommended in the individual studies, and the PTH values from different assays are not interchangeable. Frasoldati et al. [21] washed out the tissue aspirates with 1 mL saline and reported a 100% sensitivity and specificity with a cut-off level of 101 pg/mL. Using the same dilution formula, Maser et al. [23] reported that a value higher than the normal range (6–40 pg/mL) indicated parathyroid tissue and a value ranged between 49~65 pg/mL was considered questionable. Stephen et al. [19] diluted a tissue aspirate in 5 mL saline and reported a 94% sensitivity, 77% negative predictive value, and 100% specificity and a positive predictive value when the level was higher than 40 pg/mL. However, by defining the positive tissue aspirate PTH value as higher than the constant or normal PTH level, the results could potentially be contaminated if the blood is aspirated from nonparathyroid tissue and the patient has a high serum PTH [22]. Since the main source of contamination of PTH comes from the aspiration of blood, it is reasonable to define the positive tissue aspirate PTH value through a comparison with the serum PTH. Abdelghani et al. [17] washed out the aspirate with 2 mL saline and reported a 91.6% sensitivity and 100% positive predictive value when the tissue aspirate PTH level was higher than that of serum PTH at the time of performing the aspiration. Nevertheless, the dilution factor of the tissue aspirate to the saline volume was not taken into consideration in Abdelghani et al.'s [17] study and would have produced more false-negative results. In our study, the tissue aspirate was washed out into 6 mL saline, and the volume of aspirate was estimated to be no more than 0.2 mL. Therefore, a positive result was considered when the tissue aspirate PTH level was higher than one-thirtieth (0.2 mL/6 mL) of the serum PTH level. Based on this, the positive predictive value was 100%, and the presumed specificity was 100% (since the possibility of a false-positive result was nearly zero) in our series. Three false-negative results using the criterion of Abdelghani et al. [17] would yield true positive results using our criterion (case 1, 3, 28) (Table S2).

However, there are limitations to this method. To determine the negative predictive value, sensitivity, and specificity, all the assay-negative lesions should be removed. However, it is important clinically to avoid operations for the potential true negative lesions while managing persistent or recurrent renal hyperparathyroidism. One may argue that our criterion maximizes specificity without providing any evidence for sensitivity; thus, this method may offer a very high positive predictive value but also produce false-negatives. However, based on a comparison with the criteria used in other studies (Table S2), our criterion produces fewer assay-negative lesions under the absence of false positives, which justifies our definition. For the borderline assay-negative lesions (e.g., case 14, 29), repeated tissue aspiration, additional localization studies, or direct explorations should be performed. Our proposed positive assay definition is based on the assumption of the tissue aspirate volume less than 0.2 mL in the needle (0.2 mL/6 mL). Future prospective studies may be warranted to further verify this definition.

There are several strengths to this study. This is the first and largest series of tissue aspirate PTH assays performed in patients with persistent or recurrent renal hyperparathyroidism. Moreover, this is the first study to describe the complexity of pre-reoperative localization studies with uncertain or discrepant results and how tissue aspirate PTH assays could be helpful in such a difficult medical scenario. Based on the positive value of the tissue aspirate PTH assay, the relative value between the tissue aspirate PTH level and serum PTH level along with the concept of the dilution ratio was proposed to yield ideal results.

5. Conclusions

In conclusion, the selective application of a tissue aspirate PTH assay with the newly proposed positive assay definition is feasible and may help clarify the nature of suspicious neck lesions on imaging. This assay may effectively avoid negative neck explorations in patients with complicated persistent or recurrent renal hyperparathyroidism.

Supplementary Materials: Supplementary materials can be found at https://www.mdpi.com/2077-0383/10/2/329/s1. Table S1. Demographic data of patients receiving tissue aspirate PTH assays. Table S2. Comparison of tissue aspirate PTH assays results using different criteria.

Author Contributions: Study design, S.-M.H. and C.-J.H.; data collection, C.-L.H. and C.-J.H.; data analysis, C.-L.H. and C.-J.H.; manuscript writing and figure preparation, C.-L.H., Y.-C.H. and C.-J.H. All authors reviewed the manuscript. All authors have read and agreed to the published version of the manuscript.

Funding: This research received no external funding.

Institutional Review Board Statement: The study was conducted according to the guidelines of the Declaration of Helsinki and approved by the Institutional Review Board of NCKUH (A-ER-108-167) on 29 May 2019.

Informed Consent Statement: Informed consent was obtained from all subjects involved in the study.

Data Availability Statement: The data presented in this study are available on request from the corresponding author.

Conflicts of Interest: The authors declare no conflict of interest.

Abbreviations

PTH   parathyroid hormone

References

1. Yuen, N.K.; Ananthakrishnan, S.; Campbell, M.J. Hyperparathyroidism of renal disease. *Perm. J.* **2016**, *20*, 15–127. [CrossRef] [PubMed]
2. Chou, F.F.; Lee, C.H.; Chen, H.Y.; Chen, J.B.; Hsu, K.T.; Sheen-Chen, S.M. Persistent and recurrent hyperparathyroidism after total parathyroidectomy with autotransplantation. *Ann. Surg.* **2002**, *235*, 99–104. [CrossRef] [PubMed]
3. Hibi, Y.; Tominaga, Y.; Sato, T. Reoperation for renal hyperparathyroidism. *World J. Surg.* **2002**, *26*, 1301–1307. [CrossRef] [PubMed]
4. Jofre, R.; Lopez Gomez, J.M.; Menarguez, J. Parathyroidectomy: Whom and when? *Kidney Int. Suppl.* **2003**, S97–S100. [CrossRef]
5. Patow, C.A.; Norton, J.A.; Brennan, M.F. Vocal cord paralysis and reoperative parathyroidectomy. A prospective study. *Ann. Surg.* **1986**, *203*, 282–285. [CrossRef]
6. Alkhalili, E.; Tasci, Y.; Aksoy, E. The utility of neck ultrasound and sestamibi scans in patients with secondary and tertiary hyperparathyroidism. *World J. Surg.* **2015**, *39*, 701–705. [CrossRef]
7. Lai, E.C.; Ching, A.S.; Leong, H.T. Secondary and tertiary hyperparathyroidism: Role of preoperative localization. *ANZ J. Surg.* **2007**, *77*, 880–882. [CrossRef]
8. Neumann, D.R.; Esselstyn, C.B., Jr.; Madera, A.M. Sestamibi/iodine subtraction single photon emission computed tomography in reoperative secondary hyperparathyroidism. *Surgery* **2000**, *128*, 22–28. [CrossRef]
9. Irvin, G.L., III; Molinari, A.S.; Figueroa, C.; Carneiro, D.M. Improved success rate in reoperative parathyroidectomy with intraoperative PTH assay. *Ann. Surg.* **1999**, *229*, 874–878, discussion 878–879. [CrossRef]
10. Miller, D.L. Pre-operative localization and interventional treatment of parathyroid tumors: When and how? *World J. Surg.* **1991**, *15*, 706–715.
11. Neumann, D.R.; Esselstyn, C.B., Jr.; Madera, A.; Wong, C.O.; Lieber, M. Parathyroid detection in secondary hyperparathyroidism with 123I/99mTc-sestamibi subtraction single photon emission computed tomography. *J. Clin. Endocrinol. Metab.* **1998**, *83*, 3867–3871. [CrossRef] [PubMed]
12. Dotzenrath, C.; Cupisti, K.; Goretzki, E. Operative treatment of renal autonomous hyperparathyroidism: Cause of persistent or recurrent disease in 304 patients. *Langenbeck's Arch. Surg.* **2003**, *387*, 348–354. [CrossRef] [PubMed]
13. Rodriquez, J.M.; Tezelman, S.; Siperstein, A.E. Localization procedures in patients with persistent or recurrent hyperparathyroidism. *Arch. Surg.* **1994**, *129*, 870–875. [CrossRef] [PubMed]
14. Kunstman, J.W.; Kirsch, J.D.; Mahajan, A.; Udelsman, R. Clinical review: Parathyroid localization and implications for clinical management. *J. Clin. Endocrinol. Metab.* **2013**, *98*, 902–912. [CrossRef]
15. Seehofer, D.; Steinmuller, T.; Rayes, N. Parathyroid hormone venous sampling before reoperative surgery in renal hyperparathyroidism: Comparison with noninvasive localization procedures and review of the literature. *Arch. Surg.* **2004**, *139*, 1331–1338. [CrossRef]
16. Doppman, J.L.; Krudy, A.G.; Marx, S.J.; Saxe, A.; Schneider, P.; Norton, J.A.; Spiegel, A.M.; Downs, R.W.; Schaaf, M.; Brennan, M.E.; et al. Aspiration of enlarged parathyroid glands for parathyroid hormone assay. *Radiology* **1983**, *148*, 31–35. [CrossRef]
17. Abdelghani, R.; Noureldine, S.; Abbas, A.; Moroz, K.; Kandil, E. The diagnostic value of parathyroid hormone washout after fine-needle aspiration of suspicious cervical lesions in patients with hyperparathyroidism. *Laryngoscope* **2013**, *123*, 1310–1313. [CrossRef]
18. MacFarlane, M.P.; Fraker, D.L.; Shawker, T.H. Use of preoperative fine-needle aspiration in patients undergoing reoperation for primary hyperparathyroidism. *Surgery* **1994**, *116*, 959–965.

19. Stephen, A.E.; Milas, M.; Garner, C.N.; Wagner, K.E.; Siperstein, A.E. Use of surgeon-performed office ultrasound and parathyroid fine needle aspiration for complex parathyroid localization. *Surgery* **2005**, *138*, 1143–1151. [CrossRef]
20. Kim, J.; Horowitz, G.; Hong, M.; Orsini, M.; Asa, S.L.; Higgins, K. The dangers of parathyroid biopsy. *J. Otolaryngol. Head Neck Surg. = Le J. D'oto-Rhino-Laryngol. Et De Chir. Cervico-Faciale* **2017**, *46*, 4. [CrossRef]
21. Frasoldati, A.; Pesenti, M.; Toschi, E.; Azzarito, C.; Zini, M.; Valcavi, R. Detection and diagnosis of parathyroid incidentalomas during thyroid sonography. *J. Clin. Ultrasound.* **1999**, *27*, 492–498. [CrossRef]
22. Sacks, B.; Pallotta, J.; Cole, A.; Hurwitz, J. Diagnosis of parathyroid adenomas: Efficacy of measuring parathormone levels in needle aspirates of cervical masses. *AJR Am. J. Roentgenol.* **1994**, *163*, 1223–1226. [CrossRef] [PubMed]
23. Maser, C.; Donovan, P.; Santos, F. Sonographically guided fine needle aspiration with rapid parathyroid hormone assay. *Ann. Surg. Oncol.* **2006**, *13*, 1690. [CrossRef] [PubMed]

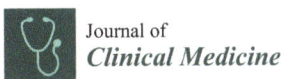

Article

Interobserver Agreement and Plane-Dependent Intraobserver Variability of Shear Wave Sonoelastography in the Differential Diagnosis of Ectopic Thymus Tissue

Zbigniew Adamczewski [1,2,†], Magdalena Stasiak [1,†], Bartłomiej Stasiak [3], Magdalena Adamczewska [2] and Andrzej Lewiński [1,2,*]

1. Department of Endocrinology and Metabolic Diseases, Polish Mother's Memorial Hospital Research Institute, 93-338 Lodz, Poland; zbigniew.adamczewski@umed.lodz.pl (Z.A.); mstasiak33@gmail.com (M.S.)
2. Department of Endocrinology and Metabolic Diseases, Medical University of Lodz, 93-338 Lodz, Poland; magdalena.adamczewska1@stud.umed.lodz.pl
3. Institute of Information Technology, Lodz University of Technology, 90-924 Lodz, Poland; bartlomiej.stasiak@p.lodz.pl
* Correspondence: alewin@csk.umed.lodz.pl; Tel.: +48-42-271-11-42
† These authors contributed equally to this work.

Citation: Adamczewski, Z.; Stasiak, M.; Stasiak, B.; Adamczewska, M.; Lewiński, A. Interobserver Agreement and Plane-Dependent Intraobserver Variability of Shear Wave Sonoelastography in the Differential Diagnosis of Ectopic Thymus Tissue. *J. Clin. Med.* 2021, 10, 214. https://doi.org/10.3390/jcm10020214

Received: 29 October 2020
Accepted: 7 January 2021
Published: 9 January 2021

Publisher's Note: MDPI stays neutral with regard to jurisdictional clai-ms in published maps and institutio-nal affiliations.

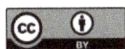

Copyright: © 2021 by the authors. Licensee MDPI, Basel, Switzerland. This article is an open access article distributed under the terms and conditions of the Creative Commons Attribution (CC BY) license (https:// creativecommons.org/licenses/by/ 4.0/).

Abstract: Shear wave elastography (SWE) has been demonstrated to be a useful tool in the differential diagnosis of ectopic thymus tissues (ETs), providing quantitative values of the shear wave stiffness (SWS) of both ETs and adjacent thyroid tissue. However, no data are available on the potential influence of the imaging plane (transverse vs. longitudinal) on the obtained SWS and shear wave ratio (SWR) values in SWE of these tissues. Moreover, no reports on the interobserver repeatability of SWE were published in regard to ETs. The aim of this study has been to evaluate the potential influence of the examination plane—transverse vs. longitudinal—on the SWS and SWR results, as well as to determine whether SWE of ETs is subjected to interobserver variability. SWE was demonstrated to have high inter- and intraobserver agreement in the evaluation of ETs and adjacent thyroid tissue. Significant differences between SWS values, but not SWR values, obtained in the transverse and longitudinal planes were observed. This phenomenon is probably a result of anisotropy-related artifacts and does not reduce the reliability of the method. SWE operators should be aware of the presence of plane-dependent artifacts to properly interpret the obtained results.

Keywords: shear wave elastography; ectopic thymus; thyroid; ultrasound; interobserver variability

1. Introduction

Ultrasonography (US) is a readily available, noninvasive tool used in neck imaging and the first step in the diagnostic algorithm of thyroid nodules [1,2]. However, US results highly depend on the interpretation and experience of the operator, with the sensitivity and specificity values ranging between 65.3 and 81.9%, and 60.7 and 68.9%, respectively [3]. Thus, some new tools based on US have been introduced for the improvement of diagnostic capabilities. Sonoelastography provides valuable information about lesion stiffness/elasticity. Malignant thyroid lesions are known to be much stiffer than benign lesions [4,5]. The first commonly available method was strain elastography (SE), which is based on a stiffness comparison of the analyzed lesion and the adjacent healthy tissue, providing the result in the form of a strain ratio only. This tool provides semi-quantitative analysis but does not allow precisely assessing the elasticity of the particular lesion. Moreover, it appeared to be researcher-dependent, as the result is associated with the degree of tissue compression [6,7]. Therefore, the use of strain elastography (SE) in US diagnosis raises much controversy. Except for supporters of this method [8], there are many opponents who do not accept the difficulties in obtaining an artifact-free result [9,10]. To avoid the limitations of SE, shear wave elastography (SWE) has been introduced. This examination is conducted without manual compression, and the result is expressed as a quantitative elasticity value (kPa). These promising properties of SWE allow us to believe that this method is accurate, operator-independent and reproducible. Such an assumption requires confirmation in the studies performed on specific tissues and organs.

Most of the studies focused on SWE concern the discrimination between benign and malignant lesions or the diagnosis of diffuse organ diseases, e.g., liver fibrosis or thyroiditis [11,12]. Only limited research has been performed to determine in vivo values for healthy soft tissues [13]. None of the published studies have included ectopic thymus tissues (ETs).

Recently, young children and even infants have been frequently referred for neck US because of enlarged lymph nodes or other palpable lumps in the neck. Ultrasound is also performed as part of a population study and due to a family history of thyroid disorders. The increasing availability of the ultrasound procedure leads to a new phenomenon of the incidental detection of various types of intrathyroidal and extrathyroidal lesions in children [14].

Any thyroid lesion found in a child should raise alertness and require further evaluation, as the frequency of thyroid cancer in thyroid lesions in children is much higher than in adults [14]. The most common benign neck lesions that can mimic malignancy are ETs [15]. The incidence of ectopic thymus in the neck in children was reported from 0.99% [16] to 1.8% [17]. Intrathyroidal ETs (IETs) and extrathyroidal ETs (EETs) resemble thyroid carcinoma and metastatic lymph nodes, respectively [15]. Proper differential diagnosis of such lesions allows avoiding unnecessary invasive procedures, including surgery. Quantitative tissue assessments in normal parenchymal organs (such as thyroid or thymus) using SWE are rarely conducted [13]. Therefore, it is remarkably important for the examiner to be familiar with normal shear wave stiffness (SWS) ranges to be able to differentiate pathological (neoplastic or inflammatory) and benign lesions.

Our research group demonstrated the usefulness of SE in the differential diagnosis of ETs [15]. However, due to the significant limitations of the method, we recently analyzed the application of SWE in children with ETs. SWE has appeared to be a useful tool in this indication, providing quantitative values of the SWS of both ETs and adjacent thyroid tissue and computing shear wave ratio (SWR), defined as a quotient of these values [18]. However, no data are available on the potential influence of the imaging plane (transverse vs. longitudinal) on the obtained SWS and SWR values in SWE of the neck tissues. Moreover, there are few studies evaluating the interobserver repeatability of SWE, and none of them include ETs or have been performed in a pediatric population [19,20].

The aim of this study was to evaluate the potential influence of the examination technique—transverse vs. longitudinal plane—on the SWS and SWR results obtained in healthy children with ETs. The aim of this research has also been to determine whether this SWE is subjected to variability between two independent researchers (interobserver variability).

2. Experimental Section

2.1. Patient Selection and Diagnostic Procedures

Fifty consecutive cytologically confirmed ETs found in 28 children who were referred to our department because of suspicion of papillary thyroid carcinoma (PTC)/neoplastic lymph nodes were included in the study. Among the 50 lesions, 33 were IETs and 17 were EETs. To exclude any thyroid disease, in all patients, laboratory tests were performed, including thyrotropin (TSH), free thyroxine (FT4), free triiodothyronine (FT3), antithyroid peroxidase antibodies (aTPO), antithyroglobulin antibodies (aTg) and TSH receptor antibodies (TRAb). All parameters were measured by electrochemiluminescence immunoassay (ECLIA) with the Cobas e601 analyzer (Roche Diagnostics, Florham Park, NJ, USA). On the basis of the laboratory results, 3 children with positive aTPO and hypothyroidism, as well as one child with Graves' disease, were excluded from the initial number of 32 children. Only children without any abnormal thyroid function and/or autoimmune disorders were included in the study. In all patients, US-guided fine-needle aspiration biopsy (FNAB) was performed under moderate sedation or general anesthesia. Cytological smears were evaluated by the same high-volume pathologist. The smears including only small lymphocytes with scattered epithelioid cells (without the presence of macrophages, plasma cells, eosinophils, histiocytes or other cell types) were diagnosed as ETs. Only lesions with cytological confirmation of ET were included in the study.

After more than 3 months from the FNAB procedure, US and SWE neck examinations were performed with a 4–15 MHz linear transducer (Aixplorer MACH30, SuperSonic Imagine, Aix en Provence, France). The neck was in a natural position to avoid hyperextension. During the SWE examination, the probe was applied gently to the skin with a gel thick coating so as to avoid direct contact between the probe and the neck. The US and SWE examinations were carried out by two independent examiners—endocrinologists with more than 10 years of experience in US and elastography of the thyroid gland (M.S.—Researcher 1; Z.A.—Researcher 2).

During the SWE examination, a single researcher performed 4 measurements in the IET group (thyroid and IET in the transverse and longitudinal planes) and 3 measurements in the EET group (EET in the transverse and longitudinal planes, thyroid in the longitudinal plane). All SWS measurements were recorded in kilopascals. SWR values were calculated for thyroid/IET pairs in both planes—longitudinal and transverse—and for thyroid/EET pairs in the longitudinal plane only, as there was no possibility to present the EET and some corresponding thyroid tissue in a single transverse plane. All children had the SWE examination carried out two times (by the two researchers) in a single session. The researchers were blinded to each other's results. No statistically significant association between patient's age and SWS of either IET or EET was previously observed [18]; thus, we did not include age into the statistical analysis.

2.2. Statistical Analysis

The analyzed variables were quantitative; they were described by the mean (as a measure of position) and standard deviation (as a measure of dispersion). Inter- and intraobserver variability of the analyzed measurements were characterized as both the absolute difference (D) and the relative difference expressed as a percentage of the absolute difference with respect to the mean value of the compared measurements (D%). Their distributions were described using the mean value together with the 95% confidence interval (95% CI). The distributions of most variables were not normal, hence the hypotheses about the equality of distributions were tested using a nonparametric method, the Wilcoxon signed-rank test. For the verification of statistical hypotheses, a value of $p < 0.05$ was considered statistically significant. To further evaluate interobserver agreement, intraclass correlation coefficients (ICC) (2, 1) were calculated, with the following interpretations: <0.40—poor; 0.40–0.59—fair; 0.60–0.74—good; 0.75–1.00—excellent [21].

All the analyses were performed using the Statistica 13.3 software (TIBCO Software Inc., Palo Alto, CA, USA).

3. Results

3.1. Interobserver Variability

The comparison between SWS and SWR results obtained by two independent researchers revealed high similarity. No statistically significant differences were found between SWS values in ETs (in IETs, EETs and both considered jointly) as well as in adjacent thyroid tissue, separately analyzed in the transverse plane and in the longitudinal plane (Table 1, Figures 1 and 2). Similarly, no differences between the researchers were found in SWR values analyzed in both planes (Table 1, Figures 1 and 2).

The ICC values computed for SWS of ETs and SWS of the thyroid in the transverse plane were 0.76 and 0.81, respectively, and 0.86 and 0.84 for the longitudinal plane, respectively.

Table 1. Comparison between SWS and SWR values obtained by two independent researchers.

	n	Researcher 1 Mean ± SD	Researcher 2 Mean ± SD	p	D Mean (95%CI)	D% Mean (95%CI)
			Transverse Plane			
SWS of ET	50	7.23 ± 1.78	7.20 ± 1.54	0.84	−0.04 (−0.37; 0.30)	10.78 (7.24; 14.32)
SWS of EET	17	6.77 ± 1.39	7.09 ± 0.99	0.18	0.32 (−0.26; 0.90)	11.26 (5.32; 17.21)
SWS of IET	33	7.47 ± 1.93	7.25 ± 1.77	0.45	−0.22 (−0.63; 0.20)	10.53 (5.89; 15.17)
Thyroid SWS	33	8.66 ± 2.42	8.54 ± 2.23	0.97	−0.12 (−0.64; 0.39)	10.49 (6.30; 14.69)
SWR of IET	33	0.89 ± 0.21	0.88 ± 0.17	0.57	−0.01 (−0.06; 0.04)	11.30 (8.01; 14.58)
			Longitudinal Plane			
SWS of ET	49	11.64 ± 3.64	12.08 ± 3.64	0.10	0.43 (−0.12; 0.99)	11.53 (7.68; 15.38)
SWS of EET	16	13.45 ± 4.30	13.99 ± 4.65	0.51	0.54 (−1.09; 2.16)	18.54 (9.67; 27.40)
SWS of IET	33	10.77 ± 2.96	11.15 ± 2.65	0.051	0.38 (0.00; 0.77)	8.13 (4.53; 11.73)
Thyroid SWS	50	11.84 ± 3.24	12.09 ± 2.85	0.36	0.25 (−0.24; 0.74)	12.86 (9.24; 16.48)
SWS of thyroid adjacent to EET	17	11.08 ± 2.57	10.82 ± 2.60	0.59	−0.25 (−1.27; 0.77)	15.57 (8.29; 22.86)
SWS of thyroid adjacent to IET	33	12.23 ± 3.51	12.74 ± 2.80	0.13	0.52 (−0.03; 1.06)	11.46 (7.23; 15.69)
SWR of ET	49	0.86 ± 0.13	0.83 ± 0.12	0.12	−0.02 (−0.06; 0.01)	9.58 (6.32; 12.84)
SWR of EET	16	0.84 ± 0.15	0.81 ± 0.19	0.51	−0.03 (−0.12; 0.06)	13.75 (6.08; 21.41)
SWR of IET	33	0.87 ± 0.12	0.85 ± 0.08	0.14	−0.02 (−0.06; 0.01)	7.57 (4.33; 10.80)

Abbreviations: CI, confidence interval; D, difference; EET, extrathyroidal ectopic thymuses; ET, ectopic thymuses; IET, intrathyroidal ectopic thymuses; SD, standard deviation; SWR, shear wave ratio; SWS, shear wave stiffness.

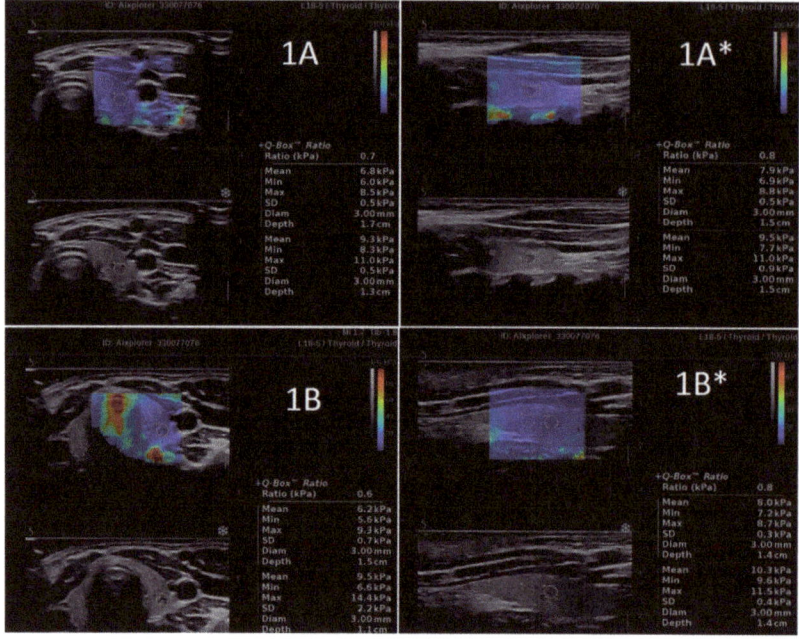

Figure 1. An example of the SWS and SWR results obtained by two independent researchers ((A) R1 and (B) R2—Patient 1. A high similarity is clearly visible for both the SWS and SWR values. * Longitudinal plane imaging. SWR, shear wave ratio; SWS, shear wave stiffness.

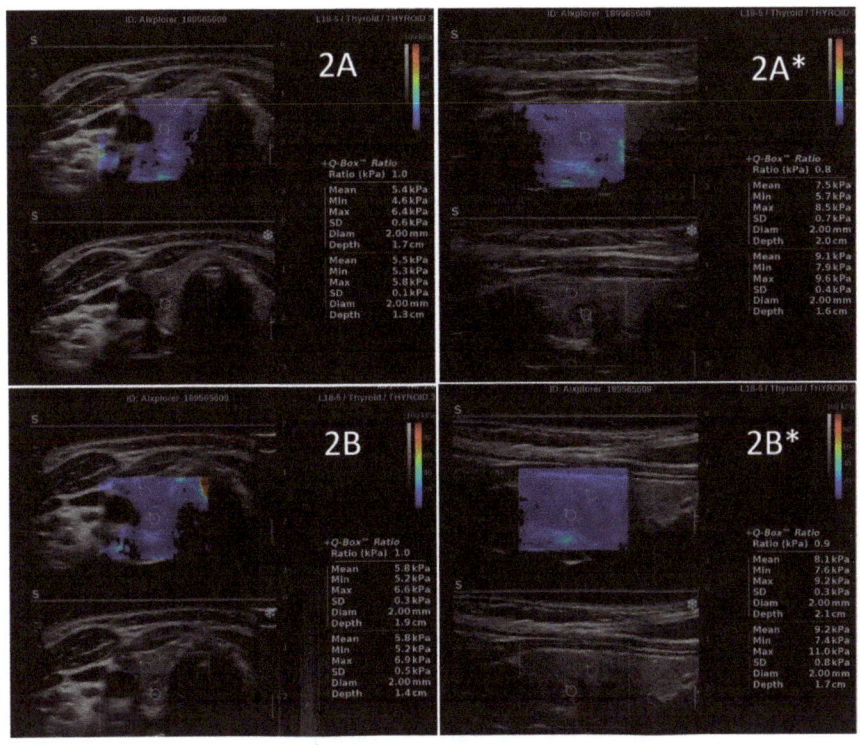

Figure 2. An example of the SWS and SWR results obtained by two independent researchers ((**A**,**B**) Patient 2). A high similarity is clearly visible for both the SWS and SWR values. * Longitudinal plane imaging.

3.2. Intraobserver Variability Related to the Imaging Plane

Highly significant differences were found in SWS values between transverse and longitudinal plane imaging. The values obtained in the longitudinal plane were higher than those observed in the transverse plane (Figure 3, Tables 2 and 3). Significant differences were found for all evaluated structures, including IETs, EETs (Table 2) and thyroid tissue adjacent to ETs (Table 3). However, no differences were found in the SWR values obtained in both imaging planes (Figures 2 and 3, Table 4).

Table 2. Comparison of SWS values of ectopic thymuses measured in the transverse and longitudinal planes.

Ectopic Thymus	n	Transverse SWS Mean ± SD	Longitudinal SWS Mean ± SD	p	D Mean (95%CI)	D% Mean (95%CI)
Researcher 1						
ETs	49	7.23 ± 1.78	11.64 ± 3.64	<0.0000001	4.40 (3.29; 5.52)	46.47 (38.08; 54.87)
EETs	16	6.77 ± 1.39	13.45 ±4.30	<0.001	6.68 (4.46; 8.90)	62.21 (48.29; 76.13)
IETs	33	7.47 ± 1.93	10.77 ± 2.96	<0.0001	3.30 (2.14; 4.45)	38.84 (28.95; 48.73)
Researcher 2						
ETs	49	7.20 ± 1.54	12.08 ± 3.64	<0.00000001	4.88 (3.85; 5.90)	47.62 (39.87; 55.37)
EETs	16	7.09 ± 0.99	13.99 ± 4.65	<0.001	6.89 (4.60; 9.17)	60.65 (47.02; 74.27)
IETs	33	7.25 ± 1.77	11.15 ± 2.65	<0.000001	3.90 (2.94; 4.86)	41.31 (32.21; 50.40)

Abbreviations: CI, confidence interval; D, difference; EETs, extrathyroidal ectopic thymuses; IET, intrathyroidal ectopic thymuses; SD, standard deviation; SWS, shear wave stiffness.

Table 3. Comparison of the thyroid SWS values measured in the transverse and longitudinal planes.

Thyroid	n	Transverse SWS Mean ± SD	Longitudinal SWS Mean ± SD	p	D Mean (95%CI)	D% Mean (95%CI)
R1	33	8.66 ± 2.42	12.23 ± 3.51	0.0001	3.57 (2.15; 4.98)	39.69 (29.86; 49.53)
R2	33	8.54 ± 2.23	12.74 ± 2.80	<0.00001	4.21 (3.05; 5.36)	40.79 (31.53; 50.06)

Abbreviations: CI, confidence interval; D, difference; SD, standard deviation; SWS, shear wave stiffness; R1, researcher 1; R2, researcher 2.

Table 4. Comparison of the SWR values measured in the transverse and longitudinal planes.

	n	Transverse SWR Mean ± SD	Longitudinal SWR Mean ± SD	p	D Mean (95%CI)	D% Mean (95%CI)
R1	33	0.89 ± 0.21	0.87 ± 0.12	0.79	−0.02 (−0.11; 0.07)	22.01 (15.57; 28.46)
R2	33	0.88 ± 0.17	0.85 ± 0.08	0.41	−0.03 (−0.09; 0.02)	13.99 (9.58; 18.41)

Abbreviations: CI, confidence interval; D, difference; SD, standard deviation; SWR, shear wave ratio; R1, researcher 1; R2, researcher 2.

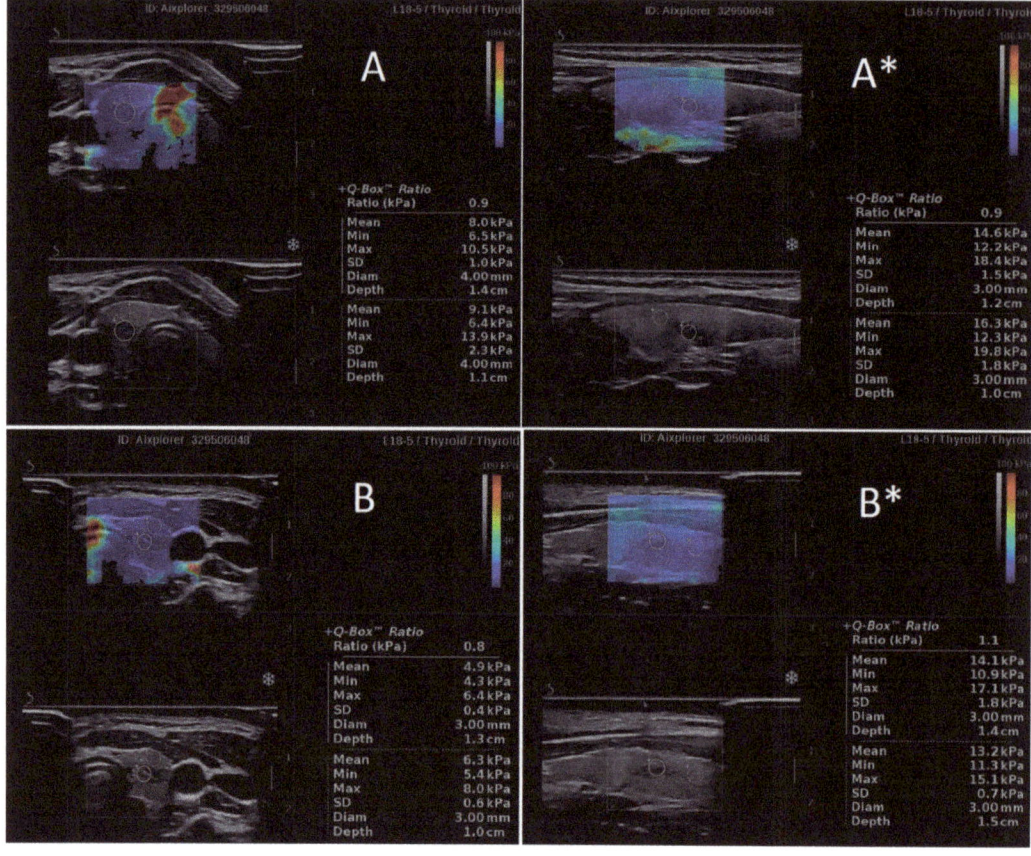

Figure 3. Examples of the significant difference in shear wave stiffness (SWS) values of two ectopic thymuses (**A**,**B**) and adjacent thyroid tissue between the transverse and longitudinal plane imaging, simultaneously with similar shear wave ratio (SWR) values, regardless of the plane. * Longitudinal plane imaging.

4. Discussion

The finding of a pathological lesion in a child's neck should arouse diagnostic alertness. Frequently, US examination is not sufficient to provide an unequivocal decision on whether the lesion is really suspicious. The differential diagnosis of ETs is an accurate example of such a situation, as benign ETs often resemble malignant lesions in US. Ectopic thymic tissues can be found in children only, and FNAB is possible to be performed in this group, mainly in sedation or general anesthesia. Thus, there is a need for an accurate, quick and simple diagnostic method for differentiation between actually suspicious lesions requiring immediate FNAB and IETs/EETs, which can be followed up for some time. In the latter case, FNAB can even be avoided in some children, especially those with some relative contraindications for anesthesia [15]. The utility of SWE in the differential diagnosis of ETs has recently been proven [18]. However, the potential influence of the imaging plane (transverse vs. longitudinal) and the interobserver variability on the obtained SWS and SWR values in SWE of the ETs and adjacent thyroid tissues has never been analyzed. Both factors can potentially modulate SWE results. Thus, the evaluation of their significance seems mandatory for the unequivocal recommendation of SWE as a reliable and researcher-independent method.

In the present study, a high interobserver agreement was demonstrated. We did not find significant differences between SWS measured by both the researchers regardless of the plane. Moreover, no differences between the examiners were found in the SWR values analyzed in both planes. A significant similarity of the SWS results was obtained in ETs (in IETs, EETs and both considered jointly) as well as in adjacent thyroid tissue. The highest difference between the SWS values reported by the two researchers reached 18.54% (EET, longitudinal plane) and was not statistically significant ($p = 0.51$) (Table 1). This observation advocates the reliability and repeatability of SWE in the diagnosis of neck structures. This high repeatability is what clearly promotes SWE over the SE technique, in which the interobserver agreement ranges from slight to fair [5,6]. Our results are not fully concordant with other reports, which provide inconsistent data. Lim et al. [22] provided results similar to ours and indicated significant interobserver and intraobserver agreement in SWE of thyroid nodules. Excellent interobserver reproducibility was also demonstrated by Veyrieres et al. [23], who evaluated thyroid nodules so as to find the SWE threshold for malignant lesions. On the other hand, in the paper by Swan et al. [24], the reproducibility of SWE of thyroid nodules was demonstrated as insufficient to reliably differentiate malignant nodules from benign nodules in an individual patient. Additionally, Kishimoto et al. [25] observed excellent interoperator reproducibility in phantoms, but it was insufficient for the thyroid and all other analyzed regions except for the liver in the healthy volunteers. Several important factors might generate this discrepancy. The most important factors are the influence of the surrounding tissues, including incorrect probe positioning (without an adequate gel thick coating, which should prevent pressure), anisotropy of the surrounding tissues, neck muscle tension or blood vessel pulsation [26,27].

In the present paper, significant differences between SWS assessed in the transverse and longitudinal planes were demonstrated in both ET and thyroid tissues. The same very high degree of statistical significance was achieved by both independent researchers (Tables 1 and 2). However, all of the obtained quantitative results measured in both planes were within the values that are considered typical for benign lesions. Chen et al. [3] demonstrated a strong difference between SWS of benign and malignant thyroid lesions, with mean values of 19.2 ± 7.1 kPa and 34.6 ± 14.8 kPa, respectively. In that group, the mean SWS cut-off level equal to 24 kPa had a sensitivity of 78.8% and a specificity of 84.9% [3]. A similar cut-off level of 22.3 kPa was presented by Samir et al. [4], with sensitivity, specificity, positive predictive values and negative predictive values of 82%, 88%, 75% and 91%, respectively. The highest SWS values obtained in our study in the longitudinal plane for IETs, EETs and thyroid tissue were 16.5 kPa, 16.6 and 22.5 kPa, respectively (, and the maximum (among the two researchers) mean SWS values in the longitudinal plane were 13.99 ± 4.65, 11.15 ± 2.65 and 12.74 ± 2.80 kPa, respectively

(Tables 1 and 2). Thus, only one highest result reached the value close to the cut-off levels, suggested by the authors cited above [3,4], and the mean SWS values were much lower than any of the cut-offs. At the same time, the mean SWS values measured in the transverse plane did not reach 10 kPa for any of the analyzed structures (Tables 1 and 2). The differences in SWS for malignant and benign lesions are particularly useful for the thyroid, as the most common thyroid malignancy is papillary thyroid carcinoma (PTC), which is distinctly stiffer than the normal thyroid tissue in SWE [11].

Despite the significant differences between SWS values in the transverse and longitudinal planes, the SWR values did not differ, regardless of the plane, and always indicated ETs as benign lesions whose stiffness was lower or equal to the thyroid stiffness (Table 3). These findings have proven that SWE is a useful method in the differential diagnosis of ETs, and the results are reliable despite the differences in SWS between the imaging planes. However, the question arises what the real reason for such differences is. To the best of our knowledge, no other publications analyzing this issue in regard to the neck structures are available, and thus we are not able to compare our results with those of other authors.

Quantitative elastography is based on the measurement of the shear wave propagation velocity and is sensitive to tissue anisotropy [27]. This phenomenon concerns tissues that have different microstructures in different planes. The shear wave speed is higher when the wave propagates parallel to the spatially oriented structures than perpendicularly to them. Therefore, when the ultrasound probe is placed parallel to these tissues, the shear wave propagates perpendicularly to them, and lower elasticity (higher SWS) values are observed. On the contrary, when the shear wave beam is emitted perpendicularly, it propagates at a higher speed, and higher elasticity values are generated. This property affects SWE values, as described before, particularly in studies concerning muscles, tendons and kidneys [27–32]. So far, this phenomenon has not been thoroughly described in the case of the thyroid gland, possibly because of the fact that the presence of anisotropy in thyroid tissue has not been confirmed on the basis of the apparent diffusion of the coefficient value in magnetic resonance examination [33]. Except for the present study, there is only one other published report analyzing SWS of the normal thyroid tissue in the two planes [34]. The authors of that paper mainly evaluated thyroid tissue altered in the course of Hashimoto's thyroiditis (HT), and the normal thyroid measurements served as controls. They reported the differences in SWS between transverse and longitudinal sections, and these differences were even more pronounced for control tissues than HT, reaching about a 40% increase of SWS in the longitudinal plane [34]. These results are highly similar to ours. Unfortunately, the authors did not make any attempt to analyze their findings.

Importantly, in our study, these differences, presented as absolute (D) or percentage (D%) values, did not differ much between researchers (Table 2). This fact can suggest that the observed difference in SWS values between the planes is actually an artifact related to the fact that most of the organs of the neck are known to be anisotropic. Such a conclusion is supported by the results of Lee et al. [26], who provided SWS values of reactive cervical lymph nodes with respect to US probe position (parallel or perpendicular to the muscle fiber orientation) and with respect to the presence of muscle stretch stress. This study revealed that SWS values were higher in the parallel position and thereby confirmed the effect of the anisotropic nature of muscles on the SWS values of the cervical lymph nodes. This phenomenon was exacerbated by the stretch stress of the cervical muscles [26].

The awareness of such a phenomenon should probably result in the indication for a mandatory description, of which a cross-section type was applied for the particular SWS measurement in the neck tissues. The possible impact of this finding on diagnosing thyroid cancers remains to be elucidated. Prospective studies evaluating SWE values in thyroid focal lesions in both planes are therefore necessary.

Thus, on the basis of the results presented in the current paper, we postulate that the elasticity measurements can be influenced by the tissue architecture of the neck organs, and this phenomenon should be taken into account when analyzing SWS results for thyroid and other neck tissues. We believe that this phenomenon should not be considered an important limitation of the method, but rather an artifact related to the physical properties of the tissues. SWE was demonstrated to be an easy and quick diagnostic method, characterized by high intra- and interobserver agreement. This might easily result in uncritical acceptance of the obtained results, while our results have demonstrated that the cross-section should be taken into account when interpreting the SWS values. Understanding the possible influence of artifacts, resulting from different plane imaging, provides the basis for eliminating errors in the interpretation of SWE.

The study has a limitation concerning the study sample calculation. ETs are uncommon findings, so the study sample was collected by including all the consecutive patients with lesions meeting the FNAB criteria of ETs, without the sample size calculation.

In conclusion, SWE is characterized by high inter- and intraobserver agreement in the evaluation of ETs and adjacent thyroid tissue. However, the researchers should be aware of the presence of plane-dependent artifacts, resulting in higher SWS values in the longitudinal section. These artifacts do not influence the SWR values and do not reduce the reliability of the method in ETs diagnosis. In our opinion, the data gained from this research will improve the diagnosis, follow-up and management of the thyroid and neck lesions.

Author Contributions: Conceptualization, Z.A., M.S. and A.L.; data curation, Z.A., M.S. and M.A.; formal analysis, Z.A., M.S. and A.L.; funding acquisition, M.S. and A.L.; investigation, Z.A. and M.S.; methodology, Z.A., M.S., B.S. and A.L.; project administration, Z.A., M.S. and A.L.; resources, Z.A. and M.S.; software, Z.A., M.S. and B.S.; supervision, A.L.; validation, Z.A., M.S. and B.S.; visualization, Z.A. and M.S.; writing—original draft, Z.A. and M.S.; writing—review and editing, M.S. and A.L. All authors have read and agreed to the published version of the manuscript.

Funding: This research was funded by statutory funds from the Polish Mother's Memorial Hospital—Research Institute, Lodz, Poland.

Institutional Review Board Statement: The study was accepted by the Polish Mother's Memorial Hospital, Research Institute Bioethical Committee (Approval Code: 45/2020).

Informed Consent Statement: Written informed consent for all the performed procedures as well as for the publication of the results was obtained from the patients' parents.

Conflicts of Interest: The authors declare no conflict of interest.

Abbreviations

CI	confidence interval
D	difference
EET	extrathyroidal ectopic thymic tissue;
ET	ectopic thymus;
FNAB	fine-needle aspiration biopsy
IET	intrathyroidal ectopic thymus;
PD	power Doppler;
PTC	papillary thyroid carcinoma;
R1	researcher 1
R2	researcher 2
SD	standard deviation
SE	strain elastography
SWE	shear wave elastography
SWS	shear wave stiffness
SWR	shear wave ratio
US	ultrasound

References

1. Dobruch-Sobczak, K.; Adamczewski, Z.; Szczepanek-Parulska, E.; Migda, B.; Woliński, K.; Krauze, A.; Prostko, P.; Ruchała, M.; Lewiński, A.; Jakubowski, W.; et al. Histopathological Verification of the Diagnostic Performance of the EU-TIRADS Classification of Thyroid Nodules-Results of a Multicenter Study Performed in a Previously Iodine-Deficient Region. *J. Clin. Med.* **2019**, *8*, 1781. [CrossRef] [PubMed]
2. Adamczewski, Z.; Lewinski, A. Proposed algorithm for management of patients with thyroid nodules/focal lesions, based on ultrasound (US) and fine-needle aspiration biopsy (FNAB); Our own experience. *Thyroid Res.* **2013**, *6*, 6. [CrossRef] [PubMed]
3. Park, C.S.; Kim, S.H.; Jung, S.L.; Kang, B.J.; Kim, J.Y.; Choi, J.J.; Sung, M.S.; Yim, H.W.; Jeong, S.H. Observer variability in the sonographic evaluation of thyroid nodules. *J. Clin. Ultrasound* **2010**, *38*, 287–293. [CrossRef] [PubMed]
4. Chen, L.; Shi, Y.X.; Liu, Y.C.; Zhan, J.; Diao, X.H.; Chen, Y.; Zhan, W.W. The values of shear wave elastography in avoiding repeat fine-needle aspiration for thyroid nodules with nondiagnostic and undetermined cytology. *Clin. Endocrinol.* **2019**, *91*, 201–208. [CrossRef] [PubMed]
5. Samir, A.E.; Dhyani, M.; Anvari, A.; Prescott, J.; Halpern, E.F.; Faquin, W.C.; Stephen, A. Shear-Wave Elastography for the Preoperative Risk Stratification of Follicular-patterned Lesions of the Thyroid: Diagnostic Accuracy and Optimal Measurement Plane. *Radiology* **2015**, *277*, 565–573. [CrossRef]
6. Park, S.H.; Kim, S.J.; Kim, E.K.; Kim, M.J.; Son, E.J.; Kwak, J.Y. Interobserver agreement in assessing the sonographic and elastographic features of malignant thyroid nodules. *AJR Am. J. Roentgenol.* **2009**, *193*, 416–423. [CrossRef]
7. Dobruch-Sobczak, K.; Migda, B.; Krauze, A.; Mlosek, K.; Słapa, R.Z.; Wareluk, P.; Bakuła-Zalewska, E.; Adamczewski, Z.; Lewiński, A.; Jakubowski, W.; et al. Prospective analysis of inter-observer and intra-observer variability in multi ultrasound descriptor assessment of thyroid nodules. *J. Ultrason.* **2019**, *19*, 198–206. [CrossRef]
8. Bojunga, J.; Herrmann, E.; Meyer, G.; Weber, S.; Zeuzem, S.; Friedrich-Rust, M. Real-time elastography for the differentiation of benign and malignant thyroid nodules: A meta-analysis. *Thyroid* **2010**, *20*, 1145–1150. [CrossRef]
9. Havre, R.F.; Waage, J.R.; Gilja, O.H.; Odegaard, S.; Nesje, L.B. Real-time elastography: Strain ratio measurements are influenced by the position of the reference area. *Ultraschall Med.* **2012**, *33*, 559–568. [CrossRef]
10. Szczepanek-Parulska, E.; Woliński, K.; Stangierski, A.; Gurgul, E.; Ruchała, M. Biochemical and ultrasonographic parameters influencing thyroid nodules elasticity. *Endocrine* **2014**, *47*, 519–527. [CrossRef]
11. Szczepanek-Parulska, E.; Woliński, K.; Stangierski, A.; Gurgul, E.; Biczysko, M.; Majewski, P.; Rewaj-Łosyk, M.; Ruchała, M. Comparison of diagnostic value of conventional ultrasonography and shear wave elastography in the prediction of thyroid lesions malignancy. *PLoS ONE* **2013**, *8*, e81532. [CrossRef] [PubMed]
12. Petzold, G.; Hofer, J.; Ellenrieder, V.; Neesse, A.; Kunsch, S. Liver Stiffness Measured by 2-Dimensional Shear Wave Elastography: Prospective Evaluation of Healthy Volunteers and Patients with Liver Cirrhosis. *J. Ultrasound Med.* **2019**, *38*, 1769–1777. [CrossRef] [PubMed]
13. Arda, K.; Ciledag, N.; Aktas, E.; Aribas, B.K.; Köse, K. Quantitative assessment of normal soft-tissue elasticity using shear-wave ultrasound elastography. *AJR Am. J. Roentgenol.* **2011**, *197*, 532–536. [CrossRef] [PubMed]
14. Francis, G.L.; Waguespack, S.G.; Bauer, A.J.; Angelos, P.; Benvenga, S.; Cerutti, J.M.; Dinauer, C.A.; Hamilton, J.; Hay, I.D.; Luster, M.; et al. American Thyroid Association Guidelines Task Force. Management guidelines for children with thyroid nodules and differentiated thyroid cancer. *Thyroid* **2015**, *25*, 716–759. [CrossRef] [PubMed]
15. Stasiak, M.; Adamczewski, Z.; Stawerska, R.; Krawczyk, T.; Tomaszewska, M.; Lewiński, A. Sonographic and Elastographic Features of Extra- and Intrathyroidal Ectopic Thymus Mimicking Malignancy: Differential Diagnosis in Children. *Front. Endocrinol.* **2019**, *10*, 10:223. [CrossRef] [PubMed]
16. Fukushima, T.; Suzuki, S.; Ohira, T.; Shimura, H.; Midorikawa, S.; Ohtsuru, A.; Sakai, A.; Abe, M.; Yamashita, S.; Suzuki, S. Thyroid examination unit of the radiation medical center for the Fukushima Health Management Survey. Prevalence of ectopic intrathyroidal thymus in Japan: The Fukushima health management survey. *Thyroid* **2015**, *25*, 534–537. [CrossRef]
17. Escobar, F.A.; Pantanowitz, L.; Picarsic, J.L.; Craig, F.E.; Simons, J.P.; Viswanathan, P.A.; Yilmaz, S.; Monaco, S.E. Cytomorphology and sonographic features of ectopic thymic tissue diagnosed in paediatric FNA biopsies. *Cytopathology* **2018**, *29*, 241–246. [CrossRef] [PubMed]
18. Stasiak, M.; Adamczewski, Z.; Stawerska, R.; Stasiak, B.; Lewiński, A. Application of shear wave sonoelastography in differential diagnosis of extra- and intrathyroidal ectopic thymic tissue. *J. Clin. Med.* **2020**, *9*, 3816. [CrossRef]
19. Grazhdani, H.; Cantisani, V.; Lodise, P.; Di Rocco, G.; Proietto, M.C.; Fioravanti, E.; Rubini, A.; Redler, A. Prospective evaluation of acoustic radiation force impulse technology in the differentiation of thyroid nodules: Accuracy and interobserver variability assessment. *J. Ultrasound* **2014**, *17*, 13–20. [CrossRef]
20. Cicchetti, D.V. Guidelines, criteria, and rules of thumb for evaluating normed and standardized assessment instruments in psychology. *Psychol. Assess.* **1994**, *6*, 284–290. [CrossRef]
21. Zhang, Y.F.; Xu, H.X.; He, Y.; Liu, C.; Guo, L.H.; Liu, L.N.; Xu, J.M. Virtual Touch Tissue Quantification of Acoustic Radiation Force Impulse: A New Ultrasound Elastic Imaging in the Diagnosis of Thyroid Nodules. *PLoS ONE* **2012**, *7*, e49094. [CrossRef] [PubMed]
22. Lim, D.J.; Luo, S.; Kim, M.H.; Ko, S.H.; Kim, Y. Interobserver agreement and intraobserver reproducibility in thyroid ultrasound elastography. *AJR Am. J. Roentgenol.* **2012**, *198*, 896–901. [CrossRef] [PubMed]

23. Veyrieres, J.B.; Albarel, F.; Lombard, J.V.; Berbis, J.; Sebag, F.; Oliver, C.; Petit, P. A threshold value in Shear Wave elastography to rule out malignant thyroid nodules: A reality? *Eur. J. Radiol.* **2012**, *81*, 3965–3972. [CrossRef] [PubMed]
24. Swan, K.Z.; Nielsen, V.E.; Bibby, B.M.; Bonnema, S.J. Is the reproducibility of shear wave elastography of thyroid nodules high enough for clinical use? A methodological study. *Clin. Endocrinol.* **2017**, *86*, 606–613. [CrossRef] [PubMed]
25. Kishimoto, R.; Kikuchi, K.; Koyama, A.; Kershaw, J.; Omatsu, T.; Tachibana, Y.; Suga, M.; Obata, T. Intra- and inter-operator reproducibility of US point shear-wave elastography in various organs: Evaluation in phantoms and healthy volunteers. *Eur. Radiol.* **2019**, *29*, 5999–6008. [CrossRef] [PubMed]
26. Lee, H.Y.; Lee, J.H.; Shin, J.H.; Kim, S.Y.; Shin, H.J.; Park, J.S.; Choi, Y.J.; Baek, J.H. Shear wave elastography using ultrasound: Effects of anisotropy and stretch stress on a tissue phantom and in vivo reactive lymph nodes in the neck. *Ultrasonography* **2017**, *36*, 25–32. [CrossRef]
27. Gennisson, J.L.; Deffieux, T.; Macé, E.; Montaldo, G.; Fink, M.; Tanter, M. Viscoelastic and anisotropic mechanical properties of in vivo muscle tissue assessed by supersonic shear imaging. *Ultrasound Med. Biol.* **2010**, *36*, 789–801. [CrossRef]
28. Otsuka, S.; Shan, X.; Kawakami, Y. Dependence of muscle and deep fascia stiffness on the contraction levels of the quadriceps: An in vivo supersonic shear-imaging study. *J. Electromyogr. Kinesiol.* **2019**, *45*, 33–40. [CrossRef]
29. Aubry, S.; Nueffer, J.P.; Carrié, M. Evaluation of the Effect of an Anisotropic Medium on Shear Wave Velocities of Intra-Muscular Gelatinous Inclusions. *Ultrasound Med. Biol.* **2017**, *43*, 301–308. [CrossRef]
30. Gennisson, J.L.; Grenier, N.; Combe, C.; Tanter, M. Supersonic shear wave elastography of in vivo pig kidney: Influence of blood pressure, urinary pressure and tissue anisotropy. *Ultrasound Med. Biol.* **2012**, *38*, 1559–1567. [CrossRef]
31. Leong, S.S.; Wong, J.H.D.; Md Shah, M.N.; Vijayananthan, A.; Jalalonmuhali, M.; Mohd Sharif, N.H.; Abas, N.K.; Ng, K.H. Stiffness and Anisotropy Effect on Shear Wave Elastography: A Phantom and in Vivo Renal Study. *Ultrasound Med. Biol.* **2020**, *46*, 34–45. [CrossRef] [PubMed]
32. Eby, S.F.; Song, P.; Chen, S.; Chen, Q.; Greenleaf, J.F.; An, K.N. Validation of shear wave elastography in skeletal muscle. *J. Biomech.* **2013**, *46*, 2381–2837. [CrossRef] [PubMed]
33. Tezuka, M.; Murata, Y.; Ishida, R.; Ohashi, I.; Hirata, Y.; Shibuya, H. MR imaging of the thyroid: Correlation between apparent diffusion coefficient and thyroid gland scintigraphy. *J. Magn. Reson. Imaging* **2003**, *17*, 163–169. [CrossRef] [PubMed]
34. Kara, T.; Ateş, F.; Durmaz, M.S.; Akyürek, N.; Durmaz, F.G.; Özbakır, B.; Öztürk, M. Assessment of thyroid gland elasticity with shear-wave elastography in Hashimoto's thyroiditis patients. *J. Ultrasound* **2020**, *23*, 543–551. [CrossRef] [PubMed]

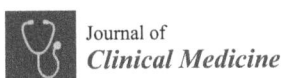

Article

Application of Shear Wave Sonoelastography in the Differential Diagnosis of Extra- and Intra-Thyroidal Ectopic Thymic Tissue

Magdalena Stasiak [1,†], Zbigniew Adamczewski [1,2,†], Renata Stawerska [1,3], Bartłomiej Stasiak [4] and Andrzej Lewiński [1,2,*]

1. Department of Endocrinology and Metabolic Diseases, Polish Mother's Memorial Hospital—Research Institute, 281/289 Rzgowska St., 93-338 Lodz, Poland; mstasiak33@gmail.com (M.S.); zbigniew.adamczewski@umed.lodz.pl (Z.A.); renata.stawerska@icloud.com (R.S.)
2. Department of Endocrinology and Metabolic Diseases, Medical University of Lodz, 281/289 Rzgowska St., 93-338 Lodz, Poland
3. Department of Paediatric Endocrinology, Medical University of Lodz, 281/289 Rzgowska St., 93-338 Lodz, Poland
4. Institute of Information Technology, Lodz University of Technology, 215 Wolczanska St., 90-924 Lodz, Poland; bartlomiej.stasiak@p.lodz.pl
* Correspondence: alewin@csk.umed.lodz.pl; Tel.: +48-42-271-11-42
† These authors contributed equally to this work.

Received: 13 October 2020; Accepted: 24 November 2020; Published: 25 November 2020

Abstract: The ultrasound (US) pattern of intrathyroidal ectopic thymus (IET) can resemble papillary thyroid carcinoma (PTC) while the extrathyroidal ectopic thymus (EET) can mimic pathological lymph nodes. Recently, the usefulness of strain elastography (SE) was demonstrated in the differential diagnosis, however this method has several limitations. The aim of the current study was to assess the usefulness of shear wave elastography (SWE) in this field. The US, SE, and SWE were performed in 31 children with 53 ectopic thymuses (ETs) and quantitative values of SWE parameters were calculated, so as to generate potential normative values of ET elasticity and of the shear wave ratio (SWR). The mean SWR_{IET} was 0.89 ± 0.21 and the mean shear wave stiffness (SWS) was 7.47 ± 1.93 kPa. The mean SWR_{EET} was 0.84 ± 0.15 and the mean SWS_{EET} was 11.28 ± 2.58 kPa. The results have proven that the stiffness of ETs is lower or equal to the thyroid's. SWE was demonstrated to be a useful diagnostic method for ET evaluation. Therefore, the application of SWE in ET diagnosis allows more accurate evaluation of ET-like lesions and, in many cases, allows one to avoid invasive procedures, simultaneously providing a precise monitoring method based on combined US and SWE evaluation.

Keywords: ectopic thymus; thyroid; shear wave sonoelastography; strain elastography; ultrasound; thyroid cancer; metastatic lymph nodes

1. Introduction

Ultrasonography (US) is an easily accessible, non-invasive diagnostic tool used in neck imaging and a first-line method for the diagnosis of thyroid gland nodules. The increasing availability of the US procedure leads to a new phenomenon of accidental findings of many thyroid and neck lesions in children. On the basis of US and postmortem examinations, the frequency of thyroid nodules in children and young adolescents/young adults was estimated at 1–1.5% and 13%, respectively [1]. The risk of malignancy in thyroid nodules in children is high, reaching 22–26%, as compared to approximately 5% in adults [1]. Thus, it is recommended to perform a fine needle aspiration biopsy (FNAB) in every thyroid lesion found in a child, except for a pure cyst [2]. Contrary to the adult population, the size of the thyroid nodule cannot be considered as an indication for FNAB in children, simply because their thyroid glands are smaller than an adult's. Thus, even small solid nodules should undergo FNAB. In children, thyroid cancer is often bilateral and multifocal, so none of these features can reduce diagnostic alertness [1,2]. At the time of diagnosis, lymph node metastases are present in most children with thyroid cancer. Hence, precise US examination of lymph nodes should be performed in every child with thyroid lesions and/or palpable suspicious lymph nodes.

In the US, intrathyroidal ectopic thymus (IET) can mimic papillary thyroid carcinoma (PTC), which is the most common thyroid cancer in children. After formation of the definitive thymus, it descends to the upper anterior mediastinum [3,4]. A disturbed process of the migration can result in ectopic thymus location, including an intrathyroidal one. The prevalence of ectopic neck thymus in children was reported as 0.99% [5] to 1.8% [6].

In the US, IETs are usually hypoechoic lesions, with punctate or linear bright internal echoes that look like microcalcifications [7]. In some cases, the lesion margins are irregular. Such features suggest PTC and require precise differential diagnosis [7]. The extrathyroidal ectopic thymic tissue (EET) is most often located very close to the lower pole of one of the thyroid lobes. Its US pattern may strongly suggest the presence of a pathological lymph node [7].

The usefulness of the strain elastography (SE) in the differential diagnosis of IETs was previously demonstrated by our research team [7]. This method evaluates tissue stiffness (elasticity) by measuring the degree of tissue deformation in response to mechanical compression [7–9]. The stiffness of the examined lesion must be compared to the adjacent healthy tissue to calculate the difference in relative stiffness. This difference is presented as a strain ratio (SR). This procedure helps to differentiate malignant thyroid lesions—which are stiffer than the surrounding thyroid tissue–from IETs, of which the SR was demonstrated to be low (0.95 to 1.09) [7]. However, SE has important limitations. Firstly, the SR result cannot be considered as absolutely investigator-independent because manual external compression in SE leads to operator-dependent variability. Secondly, the result does not provide quantitative data on the lesion's stiffness. Therefore, the usefulness of this method is limited to the lesions which stiffness can be compared to the surrounding healthy tissue. Thus, SE is useless in the case of some EETs and suspicious lymph nodes.

Shear wave elastography (SWE) is a further improvement of sonoelastography, providing a two-dimensional distribution map of tissue stiffness and quantitative measurement of the tissue stiffness in Young's modulus (kPa) and/or shear wave speed (m/s) [10]. Thus, SWE seems to be a great diagnostic tool for both IET and EET neck lesions.

The aim of the study was to demonstrate the usefulness of SWE in the differential diagnosis of ETs and to compare the results of SWE with SE. The additional aim of the study is to present US features of IETs and EETs in the largest group of cytologically confirmed ETs described so far.

2. Materials and Methods

2.1. Patient Selection and Diagnostic Procedures

Fifty three cytologically confirmed ETs found in 31 children who were referred to our Department because of suspicion of PTC/neoplastic lymph node were included in the study. Among the 53 lesions, 36 were IETs and 17 were EETs. In all patients, laboratory tests were performed, including thyrotropin (TSH), free thyroxine (FT4), free triiodothyronine (FT3), anti-thyroid peroxidase antibodies (aTPO), anti-thyroglobulin antibodies (aTg), and TSH receptor antibodies (TRAb). All parameters were measured by electrochemiluminescence immunoassay (ECLIA), Cobas e601 analyzer (Roche Diagnostics, Indianapolis, IN, USA). In all the children, US examination was performed in supine position using a 7–14 MHz linear transducer (AplioXG, Toshiba Medical Systems Corp., Tochigi-ken, Japan). Strain elastography was performed in all IET lesions (AplioXG, Toshiba Medical Systems Corp., Japan). Shear wave elastography was performed in all lesions (Aixplorer MACH30, Supersonic Imagine, France). The shear wave stiffness (SWS) and shear wave ratio (SWR) values were measured for thyroid/IET pairs and for normal thymus in transverse plane and for thyroid/EET pairs in longitudinal plane as there was no possibility of simultaneously presenting the EET and corresponding thyroid tissue in a transverse plane. All SWS measurements were recorded in kilopascals. In all patients, FNAB with US guidance was performed under moderate sedation or general anesthesia. Cytological smears were evaluated by the same high-volume pathologist. The presence of only small lymphocytes with scattered epithelioid cells (without macrophages, eosinophils, plasma cells, histiocytes, or other cell types) was considered typical for thymic tissue. The absence of lymphocytes of different stages of differentiation (as well as other cells typical for lymph nodes) allowed differentiation with lymph nodes or other lymphatic tissues. The absence of oncocytic follicular cells and plasma cells allowed exclusion of lymphocytic thyroiditis.

2.2. Statistical Analysis

The basic statistical analysis of the collected data was performed using Microsoft Excel statistical functions. Excel was also used to compute Pearson correlation coefficient values r. Statistical library scipy.stats for Python was applied to verify the correlation results and to compute the associated p-values (p). It was also used for the Mann-Whitney rank test of statistical significance between shear wave stiffness of IET and normal thymus. The p-value $p \geq 0.05$ was considered as statistically not significant.

2.3. Bioethical Procedures

In all the cases, written informed consent for all the performed procedures and for the publication of the results were obtained from the patients' parents. The study was accepted by the Polish Mother's Memorial Hospital—Research Institute Bioethical Committee, approval code 45/2020.

3. Results

3.1. Clinical Findings

The mean age of our patients was 6.91 ± 2.44 years, ranging from 3 to 12 years. The female to male ratio was 1:1.38. None of the children had any family history of thyroid carcinoma, nor any medical history of irradiation. None of the children had signs or symptoms of any relevant disease. In all patients, results of tests of thyroid hormones and thyroid antibodies were within the normal ranges (Table 1).

Table 1. Clinical characteristics of the analyzed group of children.

	Mean ± SD	Range (min–max)
Age (years)	6.91 ± 2.44	3–12
TSH (mIU/L)	2.78 ± 0.95	1.11–4.55
FT4 (ng/dl)	1.30 ± 0.14	1.05–1.56
FT3 (pg/mL)	4.11 ± 0.4	3.06–4.73
anti-Tg (IU/mL)	11.19 ± 2.89	10.0–24.4
anti-TPO (IU/mL)	11.17 ± 5.4	5.0–23.4
TRAb (IU/mL)	0.41 ± 0.2	0.3–0.91

Abbreviations: aTg, thyroglobulin antibodies; aTPO, thyroid peroxidase antibodies; FT4, free thyroxine; FT3, free triiodothyronine; TSH, thyroid stimulating hormone; TRAb, TSH receptor antibodies. Reference ranges: TSH 0.7–5.97 mIU/L for children <6 years, 0.6–4.48 mIU/L for children 6–12 years; FT4 0.97–1.67 ng/dL; FT3 2.53–5.22 pg/mL; aTPO < 34 IU/mL; aTg < 115 IU/mL; TRAb < 1.75 IU/mL.

3.2. Sonographic Findings

A total number of 53 ectopic thymic tissues were found in 31 patients. Thirty-six lesions were IETs and 17 were EETs. Ultrasound features of the analyzed lesions are presented in Table 2. The size of IETs varied from 4 to 15 mm and the mean largest dimension was 6.64 ± 2.34 mm. The size of EETs ranged from 6 to 23 mm, with the mean largest dimension of 15.59 ± 4.56 mm. Among IETs, 15 lesions were located in the right lobe and 21 in the left lobe; 22 were located in the middle part of the thyroid lobe, 13 in the lower part, and 1 in the upper part of the thyroid lobe. In six children, IET were located bilaterally, while EET were bilateral in two patients (Table 2). Coexistence of EET and IET was found in 8 children. The mean age of children with bilateral IETs was 5.83 years. The girl with the highest number of IETs (7) was 3 years old.

Table 2. Sonographic features of IETs and EETs.

	IET No. (%)	EET No. (%)
Total No. of lesions	36 (100)	17 (100)
Total No. of children with lesions	24 (NA)	15 (NA)
Shape		
• oval	21 (58)	6 (35)
• fusiform	5 (14)	1 (6)
• triangular	5 (14)	5 (29)
• round	1 (3)	1 (6)
• rhomboid	0 (0)	2 (12)
• longitudinal	4 (11)	2 (12)
Margin		
• clear	23 (64)	15 (88)
• blurred	13 (36)	2 (12)
Part of the lobe		NA
• upper	1 (3)	
• middle	22 (61)	
• lower	13 (36)	
Side		
• right	15 (42)	10 (59)
• left	21 (58)	7 (41)
No. of patients with bilateral lesions	6 (17)	2 (12)
Mean maximal size ± SD (mm)	6.64 ± 2.34	15.59 ± 4.56
• Range (mm)	4–15	6–23
Maximal number of lesions in a child	7 (NA)	2 (NA)
Bright echo shape		
• punctual	9 (25)	7 (41)
• linear	27 (75)	10 (59)
Vascularization		
• decreased	17 (47)	10 (59)
• absent	19 (53)	7 (41)

Abbreviations: EET, extrathyroidal ectopic thymus; IET, intrathyroidal ectopic thymus; NA, not applicable; SD, standard deviation.

3.3. Elastographic Findings

In SWE, the mean SWR of IETs (SWR_{IET}) was 0.89 ± 0.21, ranging from 0.5 to 1.2. Thus, the stiffness of IETs was comparable to or lower than the stiffness of the adjacent thyroid tissue (Table 3). The mean SWS of IETs (SWS_{IET}) was 7.47 ± 1.93 kPa, while the mean SWS of the adjacent thyroid tissue was 8.66 ± 2.42 kPa (Table 3). No difference between the SWS_{IET} and SWS of the normal thymus (SWS_t) was found ($p = 0.236$).

Table 3. Sonoelastographic data of IETs, EETs, and normal thymuses.

	IET SWS	Thyroid SWS	IET SWR	IET SR	EET SWS *	Thyroid SWS *	EET SWR *	EET SR *	Thymus SWS
Mean ± SD	7.47 ±1.93	8.66 ±2.42	0.89 ±0.21	0.99 ±0.13	11.08 ±2.57	13.45 ±4.30	0.84 ±0.15	0.89 ±0.13	6.96 ±1.58
Median	6.9	8.7	0.9	0.9	11.0	12.75	0.85	0.85	6.8
Minimum	3.8	4.7	0.5	0.5	5.9	6.8	0.5	0.71	4.7
Maximum	12.7	15	1.2	1.2	16.6	22.5	1.1	1.16	10.9

* EET data were collected in the longitudinal section. Abbreviations: EET, extrathyroidal ectopic thymus; IET, intrathyroidal ectopic thymus; SD, standard deviation; SR, strain ratio; SWR, shear wave ratio; SWS, shear wave stiffness.

Examples of SWE of IETs, with quantitative assessments of SWS_{IET} and SWR_{IET}, are presented in Figure 1.

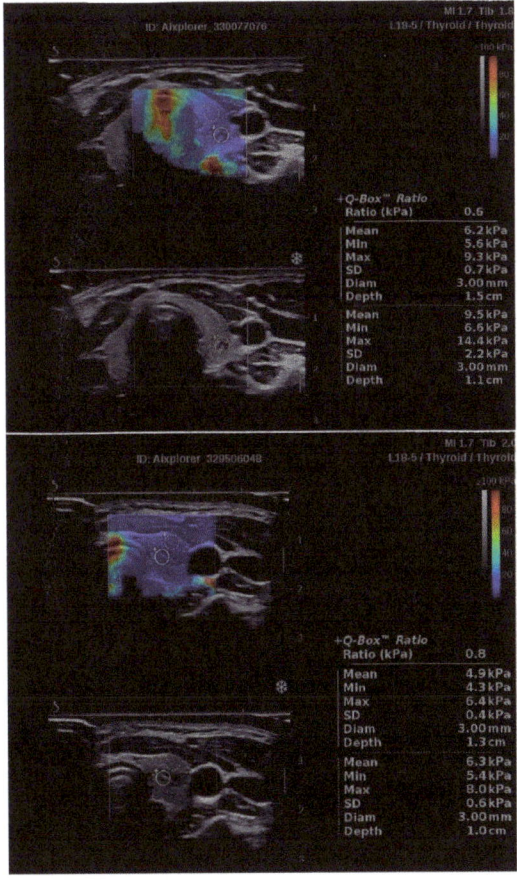

Figure 1. Examples of the application of shear wave elastography (SWE) in intrathyroidal ectopic thymuses (IETs). Quantitative assessments of shear wave stiffness (SWS_{IET}) and shear wave ratio (SWR_{IET}, described as "Ratio" in the Figure) allow one to confirm that the stiffness of the analyzed lesion is lower than the surrounding thyroid parenchyma and that the mean values of SWS_{IET} are very low (6.2 and 4.9 kPa).

In SE of IET lesions, the SR ranged from 0.5 to 1.2, mean 0.99 ± 0.13 (Table 3), which is comparable to the mean SWR$_{IET}$ result of 0.89 ± 0.21. In SWE of EETs, the comparison with the adjacent thyroid tissue was possible in 15 lesions (longitudinal section) and the mean SWR was 0.84 ± 0.15 (Table 3). The mean SR value in SE was 0.89 ± 0.13. The mean SWS was 11.08 ± 2.57 kPa (Table 1). Examples of SWE of EETs with quantitative assessment of SWS$_{EET}$ and SWR$_{EET}$ are presented in Figure 2.

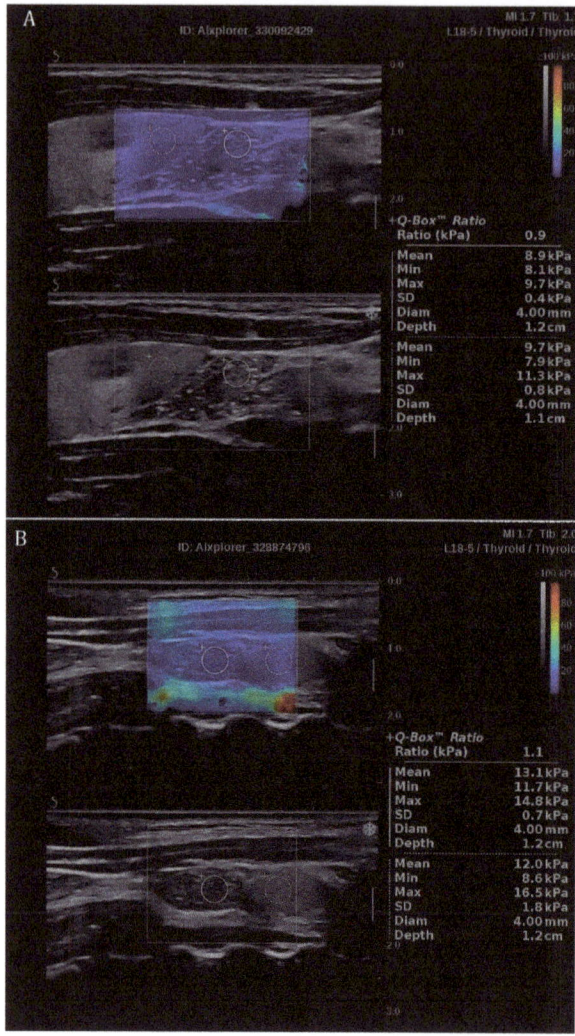

Figure 2. Examples of application of shear wave elastography (SWE) in extrathyroidal ectopic thymuses (EETs). Quantitative assessments of shear wave stiffness (SWS$_{EET}$) and shear wave ratio (SWR$_{EET}$, described as "Ratio" in the Figure) allow one to confirm that the stiffness of the analyzed lesion is lower (**A**) or similar (**B**) to the surrounding thyroid parenchyma and that the mean values of SWS$_{IET}$ are low in both of the cases—8.9 kPa (**A**) and 13.1 kPa (**B**).

No statistically significant correlation between patient's age and SWS$_{IET}$ ($r = -0.225$, $p = 0.250$) or SWS$_{EET}$ ($r = -0.029$, $p = 0.917$) was observed.

The mean SWS of the normal thymus (SWS$_t$) in the analyzed group of children was 6.96 ± 1.58 kPa (Table 3). No statistically significant correlation between SWS$_t$ and patient age was observed ($r = 0.225$, $p = 0.250$). Examples of thymus SWE with quantitative assessment of SWS$_t$ are presented in Figure 3.

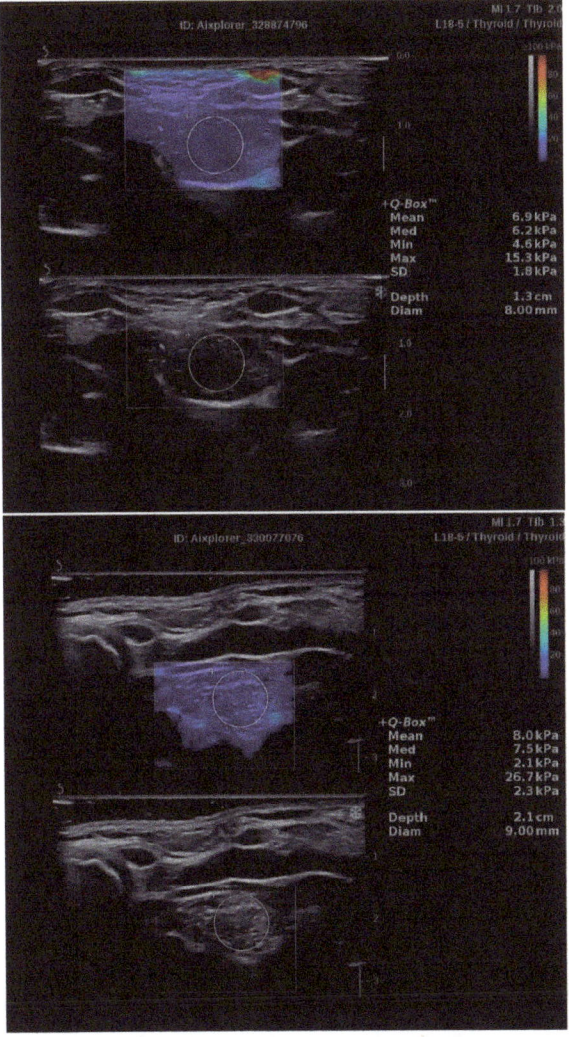

Figure 3. Examples of application of shear wave elastography (SWE) in the evaluation of normal thymus. Quantitative assessments of shear wave stiffness (SWS$_t$) reveal low values (6.9 kPa and 8.0 kPa, respectively), which are similar to those of intrathyroidal or extrathyroidal ectopic thymic tissues.

4. Discussion

The presence of a pathological lesion in the thyroid or in other cervical locations in children always arouses diagnostic alertness. IETs and EETs are frequently difficult to differentiate from potentially malignant lesions. Ectopic thymic tissues are found in children only and most of the patients are younger than 10 years of age. In this group of patients, FNAB is possible to be performed mainly in sedation or general anesthesia, which requires hospitalization. Moreover, finding a suspicious thyroid/neck lesion in a child generates significant stress for the patient and his/her parents, who need to know promptly whether the lesion may be malignant. For all of these reasons, it is necessary to find an accurate diagnostic method for a quick and simple differentiation between really suspicious lesions that require immediate FNAB and IETs/EETs, which may be observed for some time and in some cases, FNAB may even be avoided, especially if there are some relative contraindications for anesthesia.

We have recently demonstrated the usefulness of SE in the differential diagnosis of IETs [7]. Except for that paper, there is only one other published report on SE application in IETs [11]. To our best knowledge, the current study is the only one in the literature focusing on SWE in ET. Thus, comparison with other authors' results is not possible.

In the present study, we have confirmed the great usefulness of sonoelastography in ET diagnosis. SWE was demonstrated to be an accurate tool, providing a quantitative value of SWS (kPa) which is independent of any additional manual pressure required in SE. The mean SWS_{IET} and SWS_{EET} were 7.47 ± 1.93 kPa and 11.08 ± 2.57 kPa, respectively. The mean SWS_{IET} value was very similar to the SWS_t (6.96 ± 1.58 kPa). The differences in SWS_{IET} and SWS_{EET} and between SWS_{EET} and SWS_t result from the fact that SWS_{IET} and SWS_t were assessed in the transverse section, while SWS_{EET} were assessed in the longitudinal section. Therefore, SWS_{EET} values should not be directly compared with SWS_{IET} or SWS_t. The only clinical parameter that can potentially influence SWS of ETs is age as thymus tissue involution and fibrosis progresses with age. However, in our study, neither in IETs/EETs nor in normal thymus was any statistically significant association between SWS and the patients' age found. The lack of such a correlation probably resulted from the prepubertal status of all our patients. The results of SWR in IETs and in the selected EETs were 0.89 ± 0.21 and 0.84 ± 0.15, respectively. They were similar to the obtained SR values, which were 0.99 ± 0.13 and 0.89 ± 0.13, respectively. The values of SWR and SR observed in the present study confirmed our previous results based on SE, which demonstrated the SR mean value of 1.02 [7]. The only other paper published on this issue reported mean SR values in 22 IETs of 0.99 (ranging from 0.96 to 1.05) [11]. In that group, seven IETs were confirmed cytologically and 15 were diagnosed on the basis of US features. Their results together with ours—both the previous ones and the ones reported in the present paper—proved that the crucial value of sonoelastography in differential diagnosis of ETs is the fact that the stiffness of thymic tissue is lower or similar to the thyroid. This phenomenon is clearly visible on the basis of SWS values (kPa) for ET, which are lower or similar to those of the thyroid. This low stiffness is comparable to that of the normal thymus. On the contrary, the stiffness of malignant lesions is much higher than the stiffness of the adjacent thyroid and the presence of microcalcifications further increases the SWS values [12]. This is of great importance in the differentiation of IET and PTC since PTC is known to be significantly stiffer than thyroid tissue [13]. Chen et al. [14] observed the statistically significant difference between SWS of benign and malignant thyroid lesions, with mean values of 19.2 ± 7.1 kPa and 34.6 ± 14.8 kPa, respectively. The authors demonstrated that the mean SWS cut-off level equal to 24 kPa attained a sensitivity of 78.8% and a specificity of 84.9% [14]. Similar results were presented by Samir et al. [15], who reported a cut-off value for suspicion of malignancy of 22.3 kPa, having a sensitivity, specificity, positive predictive value, and negative predictive value of 82%, 88%, 75%, and 91%, respectively. The highest SWS values obtained in our study for IETs and EETs were 12.7 kPa and 16.6 kPa, respectively. These differences in SWS for malignant and benign thyroid lesions are particularly useful in the case of PTC, which covers over 90% of all thyroid malignancies in children [1]. Follicular cancer, which is often soft in elastography and different in US pattern, is extremely rare in this age group. Therefore, the usefulness of sonoelastography is of particular importance in children because it can be assumed that all lesions resembling IETs in US of which the SWS is similar to or lower than the thyroid tissue, are actually IETs. On the basis of our results and the studies by Chen et al. [14] and Samir et al. [15], we postulate to consider the ET-like lesion suspected of malignancy in the cases with the SWS value greater than 22.3 kPa (the cut-off value proposed by Samir et al. for thyroid nodules [15]).

Bayramoğlu et al. [16] have recently published a paper which provides normative values of SWS_t in regard to age and gender. In that study, the mean value of SWS_t was 6.76 ± 1.04 kPa, ranging from

4.50 kPa to 10.40 kPa [16]. Our results provide nearly identical values, with the mean SWS$_t$ 6.96 ± 1.58, ranging from 4.7 kPa to 10.9 kPa. This high consistency of the SWS$_t$ values supports that the obtained results are researcher-independent. Bayramoğlu et al. found significant negative correlations of thymus elasticity and velocity values with age [16]. However, the differences of mean SWS$_t$ between individual age groups were found to be statistically insignificant [16]. In our present study, we have not found a significant correlation between SWS$_t$ and age, although the obtained value of the Pearson correlation coefficient itself was not much lower. This probably results from the smaller analyzed number of thymuses in our study. Bayramoğlu et al. analyzed SWS values for normal thymuses only, so they could collect a much larger group of children (146 healthy children) [16].

The US-based differential diagnosis between IET and suspicious thyroid nodules is often challenging. Children with IETs are often referred for surgery as hypoechoic nodules with microcalcification-like echoes strongly resemble lesions suspicious of malignancy and cytology frequently reveals a non-diagnostic result (Bethesda category I). The application of SWE together with the detailed knowledge of the US features of ETs can highly facilitate differential diagnosis and can allow one to avoid invasive procedures in a group of children with the values of SWS, SWR, and US features typical for ETs.

Ultrasound characteristics of ETs were reported in only a few large groups of children and the IETs were diagnosed in most of them on the basis of US image only, without cytological evaluation [4,5,11,17–21]. Up to now, the biggest group with cytologically confirmed ETs was described in our previous report and included 16 lesions [7]. In most reports on the US characteristics of ETs, cytological evaluation was not performed despite the small number of lesions [3,20,21]. Such an approach carries the potential risk of misdiagnosis. Therefore, we believe that studies analyzing particular characteristic features of ETs should include lesions with cytologically confirmed ETs only.

Similarly to our previous report [7] and other studies [4,21], in the present study, the analyzed IETs were located mostly in the middle part of the thyroid lobe and less frequently, in the lower part. Having analyzed more than a three times larger number of patients than in our previous report, we found a less frequent occurrence of bilateral IETs (17% vs. 50%) [7]. This observation is more consistent with other authors' studies [3,4,21], however, on the other hand, the complete absence of bilateral lesions reported in some papers still seems confusing [6,21]. In the US, most of the IET lesions analyzed in our study were oval (58%), fusiform (14%), triangular (14%), or longitudinal (11%) in shape. The predominance of oval and fusiform IETs was also observed in other reports [7]. Oval and triangular shapes also dominated in our EET group. All the ETs were solid, hypoechoic with internal linear or, less often, punctual bright echoes. Linear echoes are easier to differentiate from microcalcifications than the punctual ones. Thus, in the cases with such punctual echoes, the application of SWE can be particularly useful as real microcalcifications substantially increase the SWS value, while the SWS of ETs remains low. Therefore, SWE can serve as a quick and easy tool to differentiate lesions suspicious for PTC or metastatic lymph nodes from ETs.

Most ETs typically have clear margins, but in some cases, the margins can be blurred, which can additionally suggest malignancy. In our present study, as many as 13 (36%) IETs and 2 (12%) EETs had blurred margins. In such US images, SWE can again clarify whether the lesion is actually suspicious.

Blood flow is known to be decreased or absent in ETs [7] and our observations are similar to other authors' findings [3–6,17–21]. In 19 (53%) of the IETs and in 7 (41%) of the EETs, no blood flow was detected. However, one should always remember that in a significant portion of PTC, vascularization can be absent and the lack of blood flow in thyroid tumors cannot be considered a benign feature [22]. Thus, once again, the application of SWE can allow us to distinguish ETs and malignancy-suspicious lesions.

It is well known that the US pattern of IETs can mimic PTCs and EETs can resemble metastatic lymph nodes. High volume experience is mandatory to distinguish the suspicious thyroid nodule from IETs in US examination. Punctual bright internal echoes in ETs are actually impossible to differentiate from microcalcifications in US. Moreover, ETs can demonstrate other suspicious US features, such as blurred margins or lack of vascularity. The awareness of typical location and US pattern of ETs is required to start with the US examination of ETs. However, in most cases, the US features do not provide unequivocal differential diagnosis. The introduction of SWE can change the quality of ET imaging as it provides quantitative assessment of the tissue elasticity and, simultaneously, it enables us to compare it with the elasticity of the thyroid. The combination of US pattern and SWE results highly improves the quality of US-based evaluation. In the first step of the diagnostic procedures, this results in the avoidance of unnecessary alert and parents' stress. In the next steps, with such an accurate diagnostic tool in the hands of an experienced ultrasonographer, this gives a chance to avoid invasive diagnostic procedures or even surgery. A typical US pattern of an ET with low SWS values may empower an experienced specialist to temporarily abandon FNAB, particularly in young children with contraindications to even short-term sedation. Regular US and SWE monitoring is mandatory in such cases.

Moreover, one should remember that rare cases of thymoma, thymic carcinoma, and lymphoblastic lymphoma arising from ET were reported [7,23–26]. Therefore, the appearance of any suspicious US feature or an increase in SWS with higher SWR always require further diagnosis.

In conclusion, SWE has been demonstrated to be a useful diagnostic method in the differential diagnosis of ETs and malignant lesions. It provides a quantitative assessment of lesion elasticity and calculates the useful SWR value by comparing this elasticity with that of the adjacent thyroid tissue. In the present study, we have provided the SWS and SWR/SR values that should be considered normative for ET. The SWS values for IETs are usually below 10 kPa and the cut-off value of below 22.3 kPa may be considered as typical for benign lesions, including ETs, irrespective of the US plane (transverse or longitudinal), provided that the SWR value is close to 1.0 or lower. Taking into account this SWR criterion is especially important if borderline SWS results are observed. SWE complements the US diagnostics and helps elucidate the suspicious US features of ETs. Therefore, the application of SWE in ET diagnosis allows for more accurate evaluation of ET-like lesions and, in many cases, helps to avoid invasive procedures, simultaneously providing the precise monitoring method based on combined US and SWE evaluation.

Author Contributions: Conceptualization, M.S., Z.A., and A.L.; data curation, M.S., Z.A., and R.S.; formal analysis, M.S., Z.A., and A.L.; funding acquisition, M.S. and A.L.; investigation, M.S. and Z.A.; methodology, M.S., Z.A., R.S., and A.L.; project administration, M.S., Z.A., and A.L.; resources, M.S. and Z.A.; software, M.S., Z.A., and B.S.; supervision, A.L.; validation, M.S., Z.A., and B.S.; visualization, M.S. and Z.A.; writing—original draft, M.S., Z.A., and B.S.; writing—review & editing, M.S. and A.L. All authors have read and agreed to the published version of the manuscript.

Funding: This research was funded by statutory funds from the POLISH MOTHER'S MEMORIAL HOSPITAL—RESEARCH INSTITUTE, Lodz, Poland.

Conflicts of Interest: The authors declare no conflict of interest.

Abbreviations

EET	extrathyroidal ectopic thymic tissue
ET	ectopic thymus
FNAB	fine needle aspiration biopsy
IET	intrathyroidal ectopic thymus
PD	power Doppler
PTC	papillary thyroid carcinoma
SE	strain elastography
SR	strain ratio
SWE	shear wave elastography
SWS	shear wave stiffness
SWR	shear wave ratio
US	ultrasound

References

1. Francis, G.L.; Waguespack, S.G.; Bauer, A.J.; Angelos, P.; Benvenga, S.; Cerutti, J.M.; Dinauer, C.A.; Hamilton, J.; Hay, I.D.; Luster, M.; et al. American Thyroid Association Guidelines Task Force. Management guidelines for children with thyroid nodules and differentiated thyroid cancer. *Thyroid* **2015**, *25*, 716–759. [CrossRef] [PubMed]
2. Niedziela, M.; Handkiewicz-Junak, D.; Małecka-Tendera, E.; Czarniecka, A.; Dedecjus, M.; Lange, D.; Kucharska, A.; Gawlik, A.; Pomorski, L.; Włoch, J.; et al. Diagnostics and treatment of differentiated thyroid carcinoma in children-guidelines of Polish National Societies. *Endokrynol. Pol.* **2016**, *67*, 628–642. [CrossRef] [PubMed]
3. Kim, H.G.; Kim, M.J.; Lee, M.J. Sonographic appearance of intrathyroid ectopic thymus in children. *J. Clin. Ultrasound* **2012**, *40*, 266–271. [CrossRef] [PubMed]
4. Kabaalioğlu, A.; Öztek, M.A.; Kesimal, U.; Çeken, K.; Durmaz, E.; Apaydın, A. Intrathyroidal ectopic thymus in children: A sonographic survey. *Med. Ultrason.* **2017**, *19*, 179–184. [CrossRef]
5. Fukushima, T.; Suzuki, S.; Ohira, T.; Shimura, H.; Midorikawa, S.; Ohtsuru, A.; Sakai, A.; Abe, M.; Yamashita, S.; Suzuki, S. Thyroid examination unit of the radiation medical center for the Fukushima Health Management Survey. Prevalence of ectopic intrathyroidal thymus in Japan: The Fukushima health management survey. *Thyroid* **2015**, *25*, 534–537. [CrossRef]
6. Escobar, F.A.; Pantanowitz, L.; Picarsic, J.L.; Craig, F.E.; Simons, J.P.; Viswanathan, P.A.; Yilmaz, S.; Monaco, S.E. Cytomorphology and sonographic features of ectopic thymic tissue diagnosed in paediatric FNA biopsies. *Cytopathology* **2018**, *29*, 241–246. [CrossRef]
7. Stasiak, M.; Adamczewski, Z.; Stawerska, R.; Krawczyk, T.; Tomaszewska, M.; Lewiński, A. Sonographic and Elastographic Features of Extra-and Intrathyroidal Ectopic Thymus Mimicking Malignancy: Differential Diagnosis in Children. *Front. Endocrinol.* **2019**, *10*, 223. [CrossRef]
8. Adamczewski, Z.; Dedecjus, M.; Skowrońska-Jóźwiak, E.; Lewiński, A. Metastases of renal clear-cell carcinoma to the thyroid–A comparison of shear-wave and quasi-staticelastography. *Pol. Arch. Med. Wewn.* **2014**, *124*, 485–486.
9. Ruchała, M.; Szmyt, K.; Sławek, S.; Zybek, A.; Szczepanek-Parulska, E. Ultrasound sonoelastography in the evaluation of thyroiditis and autoimmune thyroid disease. *Endokrynol. Pol.* **2014**, *65*, 520–526. [CrossRef]
10. Xu, H.X.; Yan, K.; Liu, B.J.; Liu, W.Y.; Tang, L.N.; Zhou, Q.; Wu, J.Y.; Xue, E.S.; Shen, B.; Tang, Q.; et al. Guidelines and recommendations on the clinical use of shear wave elastography for evaluating thyroid nodule1. *Clin. Hemorheol. Microcirc.* **2019**, *72*, 39–60. [CrossRef]
11. Januś, D.; Kalicka-Kasperczyk, A.; Wójcik, M.; Drabik, G.; Starzyk, J.B. Long-term ultrasound follow-up of intrathyroidal ectopic thymus in children. *J. Endocrinol. Investig.* **2020**, *43*, 841–852. [CrossRef] [PubMed]
12. Szczepanek-Parulska, E.; Woliński, K.; Stangierski, A.; Gurgul, E.; Ruchała, M. Biochemical and ultrasonographic parameters influencing thyroid nodules elasticity. *Endocrine* **2014**, *47*, 519–527. [CrossRef]
13. Tian, W.; Hao, S.; Gao, B.; Jiang, Y.; Zhang, X.; Zhang, S.; Guo, L.; Yan, K.; Luo, D. Comparing diagnostic accuracy of RTE and SWE in differentiating malignant thyroid nodules from benign ones: A meta-analysis. *Cell. Physiol. Biochem.* **2016**, *39*, 2451–2463. [CrossRef] [PubMed]
14. Chen, L.; Shi, Y.X.; Liu, Y.C.; Zhan, J.; Diao, X.H.; Chen, Y.; Zhan, W.W. The values of shear wave elastography in avoiding repeat fine-needle aspiration for thyroid nodules with nondiagnostic and undetermined cytology. *Clin. Endocrinol.* **2019**, *91*, 201–208. [CrossRef] [PubMed]
15. Samir, A.E.; Dhyani, M.; Anvari, A.; Prescott, J.; Halpern, E.F.; Faquin, W.C.; Stephen, A. Shear-Wave Elastography for the Preoperative Risk Stratification of Follicular-patterned Lesions of the Thyroid: Diagnostic Accuracy and Optimal Measurement Plane. *Radiology* **2015**, *277*, 565–573. [CrossRef]
16. Bayramoğlu, Z.; Öztürk, M.; Çalışkan, E.; Ayyıldız, H.; Adaletli, İ. Normative values of thymus in healthy children; stiffness by shear wave elastography. *Diagn. Interv. Radiol.* **2020**, *26*, 147–152. [CrossRef] [PubMed]
17. Bang, M.H.; Shin, J.; Lee, K.S.; Kang, M.J. Intrathyroidal ectopic thymus in children: A benign lesion. *Medicine* **2018**, *97*, e0282. [CrossRef]
18. Frates, M.C.; Benson, C.B.; Dorfman, D.M.; Cibas, E.S.; Huang, S.A. Ectopic intrathyroidal thymic tissue mimicking thyroid nodules in children. *J. Ultrasound Med.* **2018**, *37*, 783–791. [CrossRef]
19. Chng, C.L.; Kocjan, G.; Kurzawinski, T.R.; Beale, T. Intrathyroidal ectopic thymic tissue mimicking thyroid cancer in children. *Endocr. Pract.* **2014**, *20*, 241–245. [CrossRef]

20. Yildiz, A.E.; Elhan, A.H.; Fitoz, S. Prevalence and sonographic features of ectopic thyroidal thymus in children: A retrospective analysis. *J. Clin. Ultrasound* **2018**, *46*, 375–379. [CrossRef]
21. Yildiz, A.E.; Ceyhan, K.; Sıklar, Z.; Bilir, P.; Yağmurlu, E.A.; Berberoğlu, M.; Fitoz, S. Intrathyroidal ectopic thymus in children: Retrospective analysis of grayscale and doppler sonographic features. *J. Ultrasound Med.* **2015**, *34*, 1651–1656. [CrossRef] [PubMed]
22. Moon, H.J.; Kwak, J.Y.; Kim, M.J.; Son, E.J.; Kim, E.K. Can vascularity at power Doppler US help predict thyroid malignancy? *Radiology* **2010**, *255*, 260–269. [CrossRef] [PubMed]
23. Wu, S.L.; Gupta, D.; Connelly, J. Adult ectopic thymus adjacent to thyroid and parathyroid. *Arch. Pathol. Lab. Med.* **2001**, *125*, 842–843. [CrossRef] [PubMed]
24. Büyükyavuz, I.; Otçu, S.; Karnak, I.; Akçören, Z.; Senocak, M.E. Ectopic thymic tissue as a rare and confusing entity. *Eur. J. Pediatric Surg.* **2002**, *12*, 327–329. [CrossRef] [PubMed]
25. Hirokawa, M.; Miyauchi, A.; Minato, H.; Yokoyama, S.; Kuma, S.; Kojima, M. Intrathyroidal epithelial thymoma/carcinoma showing thymus-like differentiation; comparison with thymic. *APMIS* **2013**, *121*, 523–530. [CrossRef]
26. Pan, X.B.; Lang, Z.Q.; Cai, L. Primary T lymphoblastic lymphoma arising from ectopic thymus in the neck of a child. *Zhonghua Er Bi Yan Hou Tou Jing Wai Ke Za Zhi* **2011**, *46*, 159–160.

Publisher's Note: MDPI stays neutral with regard to jurisdictional claims in published maps and institutional affiliations.

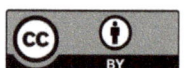

© 2020 by the authors. Licensee MDPI, Basel, Switzerland. This article is an open access article distributed under the terms and conditions of the Creative Commons Attribution (CC BY) license (http://creativecommons.org/licenses/by/4.0/).

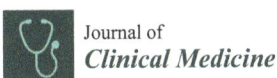

Article

Surgical Management of Primary Hyperparathyroidism—Clinicopathologic Study of 1019 Cases from a Single Institution

Jacek Gawrychowski *, Grzegorz J. Kowalski, Grzegorz Buła, Adam Bednarczyk, Dominika Żądło, Zbigniew Niedzielski, Agata Gawrychowska and Henryk Koziołek

Department of General and Endocrine Surgery, Faculty of Medical Sciences in Zabrze, Medical University of Silesia, 40-055 Katowice, Poland; kowalskigrzeg@gmail.com (G.J.K.); gregor6007@onet.eu (G.B.); adambednarczyk90@gmail.com (A.B.); dominika.zadlo@gmail.com (D.Ż.); zbigniew.niedzielski@wp.pl (Z.N.); agatagawrychowska86@gmail.com (A.G.); henkoz@interia.pl (H.K.)
* Correspondence: chirurgiabytom@sum.edu.pl

Received: 24 September 2020; Accepted: 28 October 2020; Published: 2 November 2020

Abstract: Background: Primary hyperparathyroidism (pHPT) is an endocrine disorder characterized by hypercalcemia and caused by the presence of disordered parathyroid glands. Parathyroidectomy is the only curative therapy for pHPT, but despite its high cure rate of 95–98%, there are still cases where hypercalcemia persists after this surgical procedure. The aim of this study was to present the results of a surgical treatment of patients due to primary hyperparathyroidism and failures related to the thoracic location of the affected glands. Methods: We present a retrospective analysis of 1019 patients who underwent parathyroidectomy in our department in the period 1983–2018. Results: Among the group of 1019 operated-on patients, treatment failed in 19 cases (1.9%). In 16 (84.2%) of them, the repeated operation was successful. In total, 1016 patients returned to normocalcemia. Conclusions: Our results confirm that parathyreoidectomy is the treatment of choice for patients with primary hyperparathyroidism. The ectopic position of the parathyroid gland in the mediastinum is associated with an increased risk of surgical failure. Most parathyroid lesions in the mediastinum can be safely removed from the cervical access.

Keywords: primary hyperparathyroidism; parathyroidectomy; remedial surgery; ectopic mediastinal localization; persistent hypercalcemia

1. Introduction

Primary hyperparathyroidism (pHPT) is a type of endocrine disorder resulting in increased secretion of the parathyroid hormone from abnormal parathyroid glands. It leads to serious disturbances in calcium and phosphate metabolism leading to elevated levels of calcium in blood serum which may be a risk factor for developing a hypercalcemic crisis [1,2]. Primary hyperparathyroidism is a relatively common disorder that is diagnosed in 0.1 to 1% of the general population, and more often in postmenopausal women [2]. In patients with pHPT, the parathormone (PTH) excess originates from neoplastic or hyperplastic cells of parathyroid parenchyma. Most cases involved a single abnormal parathyroid gland located in an usual neck site, but many of such changes occur in other sites including the thymus gland, the retroesophageal space or the thyroid gland. Sometimes, parathyroid lesions have been reported in the pericardium or soft and adipose tissues of the mediastinum up to the angle of the jaw [3,4]. The differentiation between hyperplasia and adenoma may not be easy even for an experienced surgeon. In case of hyperplasia, it is essential to the establish not only the size, but also the symmetry of affected glands. In many cases, even affected glands can appear normal in the gross appearance. This points to the importance of a biopsy taken from the tissue and its examination by a pathologist. Parathyroidectomy (PTX) is the procedure of choice for patients suffering from pHPT with a cure rate of 95–98%. Such an operation is now the procedure of choice at experienced surgical centers, with the use of an intraoperative PTH level (iPTH). However, even then the PTX for ectopic mediastinal lesions is a challenging procedure [4]. We reported a group of 1019 patients operated on for pHPT between the years 1983 and 2018.

2. Materials and Methods

This is a retrospective study of 1019 patients operated on between 1983 and 2018 (between 1983 and 2004 318 patients were operated on and from 2005 to 2018 701 patients were operated on) (Figure 1) for primary hyperparathyroidism (pHPT). The sample consisted of 759 women (74.5%) and 260 men (25.5%) between the ages of 19 and 81. We evaluated 953 operated-on patients during the same time period for parathyroid lesions located in the neck and carried out comparisons with a group of 66 patients with ectopic mediastinal lesions. Patients were identified based on operation protocols and histopathological findings regarding the number of lesions, their localization, and biochemical and surgical results. The diagnostic management consisted of a careful case history and physical examination, and routine biochemical examinations. The biochemical examinations included measurements of the serum calcium levels and intact PTH. Parathyroid localization studies included up until 2004 the ultrasound and subtraction technique (also known as dual-isotope imaging); from 2005 sestamibi technetium-99 m scintigraphy was used and from 2010, the single-photon emission computed tomography (SPECT) technique has usually been utilized, and rarely the CT scan. Two positive imaging studies were always required. Upon their discharge from the hospital, the patients were seen at least four times a year—i.e., every three months within the first two years and every six months thereafter. Physical and biochemical examinations were also performed. We arbitrarily divided cases of hypercalcemia after prior surgery into persistent (defined as hypercalcemia recurring within six months of the initial operation) or recurrent (hypercalcemia recurring after six months of normocalcemia).

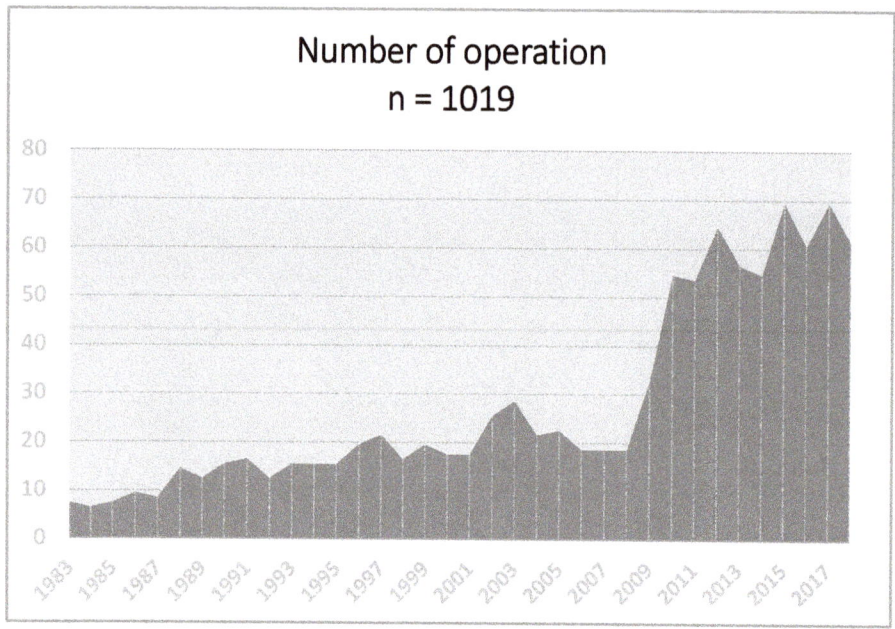

Figure 1. Number of operations in years 1983–2018.

3. Methods of Statistical Analysis

All of the collected data were included in a spreadsheet in Microsoft Office Excel 2019. The statistical analysis was performed in Statistica 12.5. After establishing and classifying the data using a Kolmogorow–Smirnow test, we used a Student's t-test to compare data with a normal distribution and for the data non-normal distribution we used the Mann–Whitney U test. The results are presented as percentage changes, full numbers, means and standard deviations. The numerical data were compared with that of the Pearson chi-square test. The level of significance was calculated at $p < 0.05$. Effect size—ES—was determined using Youle's Phi coefficient and Cramer's V.

4. Results

Parathyroid lesions were identified in 1019 patients. Fatigue, muscle or bone weakness, and loss of appetite were the most commonly observed symptoms in 923 symptomatic patients with normal or ectopic localizations of dysfunctional parathyroid glands. No symptoms were recorded among the remaining 96 patients (Table 1).

Table 1. Symptoms of 1019 patients operated on for Primary hyperparathyroidism (pHPT).

Symptom or Sign	Whole Group of Patients ($n = 1019$)	Patients with Neck Localization ($n = 953$)	Patients with Mediastinal Localization ($n = 66$)	χ^2	p Value	φ
Bone and muscle pain	797 (78.4%)	750 (78.7%)	47 (71.2%)	2.03	0.154	0.05
Arterial hypertension	493 (48.5%)	480 (50.4%)	13 (19.7%)	23.25	<0.001	0.15
Nephrolithiasis	385 (37.9%)	359 (37.7%)	26 (39.4%)	0.08	0.780	0.01
Osteoporosis	245 (24.1%)	229 (24%)	16 (24.2%)	<0.01	0.969	<0.01
Fatigue	242 (23.8%)	227 (23.8%)	15 (22.7%)	0.04	0.840	<0.01
Constipation	226 (22.2%)	211 (22.1%)	15 (22.7%)	0.01	0.912	<0.01
Mental depression	162 (15.9%)	152 (15.9%)	10 (15.2%)	0.03	0.864	<0.01
Chronic renal insufficiency	145 (14.3%)	153 (16.1%)	9 (13.6%)	0.27	0.603	0.02
Weight loss	129 (12.7%)	121 (12.7%)	8 (12.1%)	0.02	0.892	<0.01
Stomach ulcer/Duodenal ulcer	113 (11.1%)	106 (11.1%)	7 (10.6%)	0.02	0.897	<0.01
Pathological bone fracture	97 (9.5%)	91 (9.5%)	6 (9.1%)	0.02	0.902	<0.01
Acute or chronic pancreatitis	80 (7.9%)	75 (7.9%)	5 (7.6%)	<0.01	0.932	<0.01
Loss of appetite	275 (27%)	261 (27.4%)	14 (21.2%)	1.20	0.274	0.03
Dermatopathies	32 (3.1%)	23 (2.4%)	9 (13.6%)	25.56	<0.001	0.16
Without symptoms	96 (9.4%)	92 (9.7%)	4 (6.1%)	0.93	0.334	0.03

The vast majority (93.6%) of parathyroid lesions were localized in the neck (predominantly within the left and right superior glands), whereas a minority (6.4%) were found in the mediastinum. We observed a significant difference in the occurrence of arterial hypertension among the patients with neck parathyroid glands when compared to mediastinal localization. Dermopathies were significantly more frequent in the group of patients operated on for mediastinal glands, but both effect sizes were weak.

Histological findings demonstrated benign lesions in 990 patients while malignancy was reported in the remaining 29 cases. Among the 1019 patients, we investigated 1226 lesions, with 856 of them related to a single gland and 163 impacting two or more glands (Table 2). Among multiple lesions, the affection of two glands was the most prominent, while affection of four glands was sporadic. The benign neoplasms have been further differentiated into hyperplasia—which were identified most often (827 lesions)—and adenomas, which made up the remaining 370 lesions.

Table 2. Patient's characteristics.

Factor			No. of Patients/Localization			p Value	ES
			All $n = 1019$	Neck $n = 953$	Mediastinum $n = 66$		
sex		M	260	244	16	0.806	0.01
		F	759	709	50		
age (years)		M	21–79 (55.0)	21–79 (55.0)	25–79 (55.9)	0.240	0.01
		F	19–81 (55.0)	19–81 (55.4)	28–80 (56.2)	0.339	<0.01
symptoms		Yes	923	861	62	0.334	0.03
		No	96	92	4		
lesion		benign	990	928	62	0.104	0.05
		malignant	29	25	4		
no. of lesions		single	856	807	49	0.070	0.08
		multiple	163	146	17		
		2	129	114	15		
		3	26	24	2		
		4	8	8	0		
localization	left	superior	220	210	10	0.015	0.10
		inferior	351	315	36		
	right	superior	219	213	6	0.014	0.10
		inferior	436	403	33		
histopathology $n = 1226$		hyperplasia	827	772	55	0.460	0.05
		adenoma	370	344	26		
		cancer	29	25	4		
Recurrent nerve palsy			11	7	4	<0.001	0.2
		transient	9	7	2		
		permanent	2	0	2		
Operation failure			19 (1.7%)	8 (0.8%)	11 (16.7%)	<0.001	0.26

The analysis of biochemical examination results indicated elevated serum calcium and parathyroid hormone levels within the entire group prior to operation without distinction of etiologies or localizations (Figures 2 and 3).

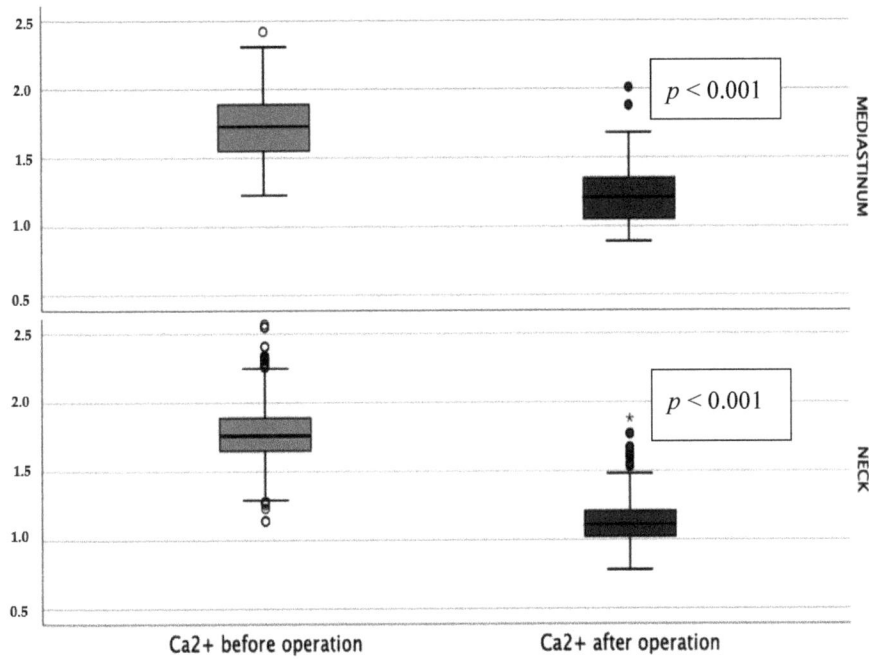

Figure 2. Blood serum Ca^{2+} concentration before and after operation (*—$p < 0.001$).

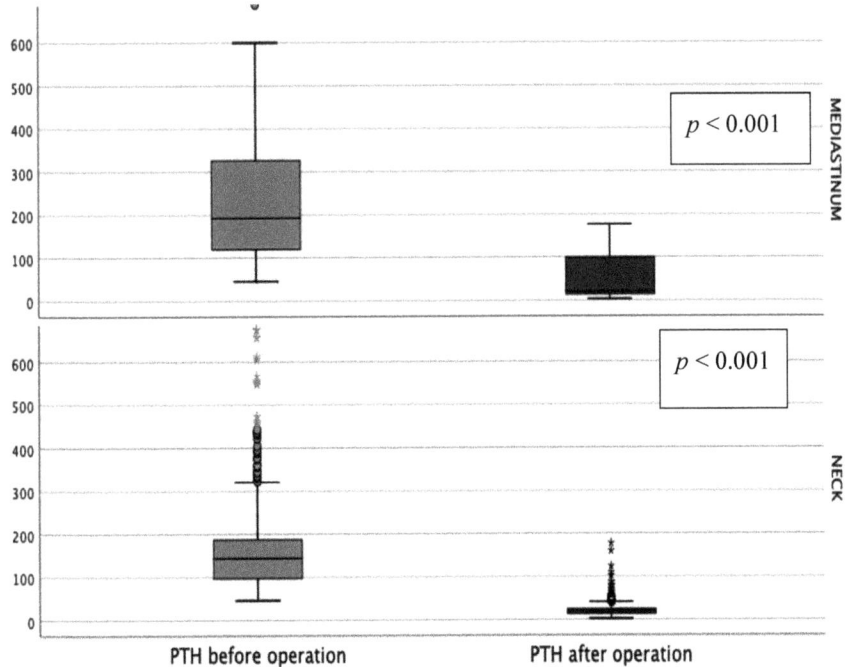

Figure 3. Blood serum parathormone (PTH) concentration before and after operation (*—$p < 0.001$).

Histopathological findings imply that hyperplasia and adenoma are the most common types of single and multiple lesions (Table 3). In the case of multiple lesions, the intercurrence of adenoma and hyperplasia of several glands occurred within the neck area, but it was not seen in mediastinal localization.

Table 3. Histopathological findings.

Number of Affected Parathyroid Glands	Histopathological Finding	Patients/Abnormalities			χ^2	p Value	φ
		All	Neck	Mediastinum			
Single	Hyperplasia	492	464	28	2.44	0.486	0.05
	Adenoma	337	319	18			
	Cancer	27	24	3			
	All	856	807	49			
Two or More	2 × hyperplasia + cancer	1	1	0	0.07	0.792	<0.01
	1 × hyperplasia + cancer	1	0	1	14.45	<0.001	0.12
	2 × hyperplasia	82	73	9	2.98	0.084	0.05
	2 × adenoma	8	5	3	12.81	<0.001	0.11
	3 × hyperplasia	20	18	2	0.42	0.518	0.02
	hyperplasia + adenoma	36	34	2	0.05	0.819	<0.01
	4 × hyperplasia	5	5	0	0.35	0.560	<0.01
	2 × hyperplasia + adenoma	6	6	0	0.42	0.520	<0.01
	3 × hyperplasia + adenoma	3	3	0	0.21	0.648	<0.01
	2 × adenoma + hyperplasia	1	1	0	0.07	0.792	<0.01
	sum	163	146	17	5.00	0.025	0.07

During performing operations, we discovered that the parathyroid gland most commonly affected within the entire group of patients was the inferior right, with 436 cases. The inferior left parathyroid gland was affected in 351 cases, superior left in 220 cases, and superior right in 219 cases. We also performed a comparison of the occurrence of neoplastic gland in patients with single-gland changes and those with multiple abnormal glands. In the case of patients with single-gland neoplasm, the most commonly affected was the inferior right parathyroid gland (347 cases) and subsequently the superior left (142 cases), the superior right (140 cases), and the inferior left (27 cases). Within the patients with more than one affected gland, abnormalities were found most often within the inferior right parathyroid gland (89 cases) and subsequently the superior right (79 cases), the superior left (78 cases), and rarely the inferior left parathyroid gland (24 cases). Double adenomas were situated most commonly in the lower right location (53%), subsequently the right (49%) and the upper left (30%) locations, and sporadically in the lower left location (17%), implying that double adenomas are usually found in the right part of the neck when parathyroid glands are not ectopic. The mean size of double adenomas was approximately 1.5 cm. After a parathyroidectomy was performed, no symptoms were prominent among almost all of the patients and both PTH and calcium levels decreased. Calcium levels has normalized postoperatively and remained within the normal range for 12 months or longer.

A total of 19 patients required remedial surgery due to persistent or recurrent hypercalcemia. Out of the group of 1019 patients, failures in the surgical treatment of pHPT were reported in 19 cases—in eight cases, the lesions were located on the neck, and in 11 cases the lesions were in the mediastinum (Table 4).

Table 4. Treatment failures.

Localization	Number of Patients	Treatment Failures	χ^2	p Value	φ
All	1019	19 (1.9%)			
Neck	953	8 (0.8%)	21.15	<0.001	0.15
Mediastinum	66	11 (16.6%)			

Persistent hyperfunction was the cause of repeated operation in nine of them and relapse in 10. However, imaging studies failed to find the cause of the hyperfunction in three of them. The remaining 16 were operated on successfully (Table 5).

Table 5. Persistent and recurrent hypercalcemia.

Localization	Number of Patients	Hypercalcemia		Changes Not Found	χ^2	p Value	φ
		Persistent	Recurrent				
All	1019	9 (0.9%)	7 (0.7%)	3 (0.3%)			
Neck	953	2 (0.2%)	4 (0.4%)	2 (0.2%)	2.05	0.152	0.36
Mediastinum	66	7 (10.6%)	3 (4.5%)	1 (1.5%)			

There were two (0.2%) cases of persistent hypercalcemia caused by lesions of the neck and some cases (10.6%) in the mediastinum. Recurrent hypercalcemia was found in four patients (0.4%) due to a neoplastic gland remaining in the neck area and three (4.5%) within the mediastinum. We did not find any changes in three cases, where two cases were related to a neck localization and one case to the mediastinum. The main cause of failure of the surgical treatment were parathyroid carcinomas (twice—the cause of persistent activity and four—recurrent).

5. Discussion

Parathyroidectomy is the treatment of choice in patients with primary hyperparathyroidism. The goal of PTX is to achieve normocalcemia by removal of the hyperfunctioning tissue that causes excessive secretion of parathyroid hormones. Surgical failures may result from an incomplete excision or parathyromatosis. Reoperative parathyroid surgery can be required in approximately 10% of patients [5]. Out of the 1019 patients, 19 (1.9%) received a surgery that failed. This mainly applies to patients with ectopic mediastinal lesions (16.6%).

We want to emphasize that 15% of our patients have a multiple gland disease and that the heterogenic group includes patients with multiple hyperplasia, double adenoma, hyperplasia as well as cancer. We believe that a visual indication of all parathyroid glands and excision or biopsy of the rest of them is an effective procedure for most patients operated on for pHPT. Moreover, in our opinion, an intraoperative measurement of PTH (iPTH) by a quick assay (QPTH) in predicting operative outcomes of parathyroidectomy is the procedure of choice. For the last 15 years we have measured QPTH in all operated-on patients. The goal of the surgical treatment is to remove hyperfunctioning glands. If hyperplasia is diagnosed, we remove three and a half parathyroid glands, or hyperfunctioning adenomas. Collar incision is a feasible approach to the mediastinal glands even at re-exploration. Among our 66 patients treated for a mediastinal ectopic gland, only four required thoracotomy. We must emphasize that about one-third of normal lower parathyroid glands are found below the lower thyroid pole, in the thyroid-thymic tract of fat or cervical tongue of the thymus. In our experience of reoperation for a "missing" gland, the thymus is its most probable location. Among seven of our patients reoperated on for persistent hypercalcemia, four glands were found within the thymus, one between the pericardial sac and the mediastinal pleura, close to the main left bronchus, one in the aorto-pulmonary window and one close to the right innominate vein and the superior vena cava.

The analysis of surgical treatment failures for various parathyroid changes implies several explanations. These include the variable anatomy of parathyroid glands among different patients as well as ectopic locations of adenomas [6]. There are various opinions that all glands inferior to the superior border of the manubrium tend to be mediastinal [6,7]. Others consider that mediastinal parathyroid glands are those which are unreachable by cervical incisions [7,8]. On the other hand, we noted an extreme case where the changed parathyroid gland appeared in the soft palate of a 57-year old patient who suffered from persistent hypercalcemia even after initial parathyroidectomy. The investigation of this patient also shows that there is still a possibility that parathyroid adenomas can be missed even with previous use of advanced imaging methods if they occur in various anatomical positions [9]. Moreover, ectopic parathyroid glands can be so small that they may be invisible, or a single removed gland is one when all function abnormally [5,7]. In our opinion, the best surgical solution for the latter is a removal of three and a half of the parathyroid glands. Re-operation is also required when one of two affected glands is more active than the other. In such a situation, when the dominant parathyroid gland has been removed, the other becomes the cause of hyperfunction. A second operation is also needed when the altered parathyroid gland has not been completely removed—for example, when undergoing disintegration—and the rest of the parathyroid gland develops again causing symptoms of hyperactivity.

Most of the reasons for the failure of initial parathyroidectomy may be eliminated by the right diagnostic measures in the form of imaging possibilities [10,11]. Radiological examination methods are particularly precise and helpful to properly localize most of hyperfunctioning parathyroid glands, thus allowing for shorter surgeries, a decrease in ineffective surgeries and fewer complications [12,13]. Some studies show that in primary hyperparathyroidism the results of preoperative imaging examinations do not allow to differentiate between a uniglandular and multiglandular disease in [14,15]. Finding the parathyroid gland facilitates the intraoperative examination of parathyroid hormone concentration, as well as the use of radio-guidance [16–18].

Cases with multiple tumours are particularly more complicated, as a fall in the intraoperative PTH to the lower end of a normal range cannot guarantee that all tumours have been removed [19–21]. A reduction in intraoperative PTH by more than 50% after the procedure is a predictive factor [22,23] and may be prevented by preoperative supplementation with bisphosphonates [24,25]. Age is not a relevant contributing factor for the occurrence of complications [26,27], while anesthesia can often cause sudden elevation of PTH levels in patients suffering from hyperparathyroidism [28,29] and can worsen renal functions [30,31]. The latest works shows that minimally invasive radio-guided parathyroidectomy using a very low dose of Tc-99 MIBI, even without an intraoperative assay or a frozen section analysis, resulted in an excellent cure rate [32,33]. Based on our results, we also wanted to emphasize that PTX is a safe procedure, with only a small number of complications, the most serious of which seems to be recurrent laryngeal nerve palsy. Based on our observations, we believe that patients should be examined every three months after PTX for the first two years, and then twice a year afterwards. Some authors indicate that this should last for even more than 10 years after parathyroidectomy [34].

6. Conclusions

(1) Our results confirm that parathyroidectomy is the treatment of choice in patients with primary hyperparathyroidism.
(2) Ectopic position of the parathyroid gland in the mediastinum is associated with an increased risk of surgical failure.
(3) Most parathyroid lesions in the mediastinum can be safely removed from the cervical access.

Author Contributions: Conceptualization, J.G.; Methodology, G.B., A.B., D.Ż., Z.N., A.G. and H.K.; Writing—original draft, G.J.K. All authors have read and agreed to the published version of the manuscript.

Funding: This research received no external funding.

Conflicts of Interest: The authors declare no conflict of interest.

References

1. Sahli, Z.T.; Karipineni, F.; Zeiger, M.A. A garden of parathyroid adenomas. *BMJ Case Rep.* **2017**, *2017*, bcr-2017. [CrossRef] [PubMed]
2. Al-Sobhi, S.; Clark, O.H. Parathroid hyperplasia; Parathroidectomy. In *Textbook of Endocrine Surgery*, 1st ed.; Clark, O.H., Duh, Q.Y., Eds.; WB Saunders Company: Philadelphia, PA, USA, 1997; pp. 372–379.
3. Uludag, M.; Aygün, N.; Isgor, A. Main Surgical Principles and Methods in Surgical Treatment of Primary Hyperparathyroidism. *SiSli Etfal Häst. Tip Bul.* **2019**, *53*, 337–352.

4. Kowalski, G.J.; Bula, G.; Zadlo, D.; Gawrychowska, A.; Gawrychowski, J. Primary Hyperparathyroidism. *Endokrynol. Pol.* **2020**, *71*, 260–270. [CrossRef] [PubMed]
5. Stack, B.C., Jr.; Tolley, N.S.; Bartel, T.B.; Bilezikian, J.P.; Bodenner, D.; Camacho, P.; Cox, J.P.D.T.; Dralle, H.; Jackson, J.E.; Morris, J.C.; et al. AHNS Series: Do you know your guidelines? Optimizing outcomes in reoperative parathyroid surgery: Definitive multidisciplinary joint consensus guidelines of the American Head and Neck Society and the British Association of Endocrine and Thyroid Surgeons. *Head Neck* **2018**, *40*, 1617–1629. [CrossRef] [PubMed]
6. Navarro, A.; Vassallo, J.; Galea, J. Excision of an Elusive Tiny Ectopic Parathyroid Adenoma. *Case Rep. Oncol.* **2017**, *10*, 1105–1111. [CrossRef]
7. Sunny, S.A.; Singh, A.; Adhikary, A.B. Ectopic Parathyroid Adenoma: Surgical Correction and its Complication Management. *Mymensingh Med. J. MMJ* **2019**, *28*, 245–249.
8. Chang, B.A.; Sharma, A.R.; Anderson, D.W. Ectopic parathyroid adenoma in the soft palate: A case report. *J. Otolaryngol. Head Neck Surg.* **2016**, *45*, 53. [CrossRef]
9. Madsen, A.R.; Rasmussen, L.; Godballe, C. Risk factors for treatment failure in surgery for primary hyperparathyroidism: The impact of change in surgical strategy and training procedures. *Eur. Arch. Oto-Rhino-Laryngology* **2015**, *273*, 1599–1605. [CrossRef]
10. Van Udelsman, B.; Udelsman, R. Surgery in Primary Hyperparathyroidism: Extensive Personal Experience. *J. Clin. Densitom.* **2013**, *16*, 54–59. [CrossRef]
11. Kazaure, H.S.; Thomas, S.; Scheri, R.P.; Stang, M.; Roman, S.A.; Sosa, J.A. The devil is in the details: Assessing treatment and outcomes of 6,795 patients undergoing remedial parathyroidectomy in the Collaborative Endocrine Surgery Quality Improvement Program. *Surgery* **2019**, *165*, 242–249. [CrossRef]
12. Untch, B.R.; Adam, M.A.; Danko, M.E.; Barfield, M.E.; Dixit, D.; Scheri, R.P.; Olson, J.A. Tumor Proximity to the Recurrent Laryngeal Nerve in Patients with Primary Hyperparathyroidism Undergoing Parathyroidectomy. *Ann. Surg. Oncol.* **2012**, *19*, 3823–3826. [CrossRef]
13. Patel, S.G.; Saunders, N.D.; Jamshed, S.; Weber, C.J.; Sharma, J. Multimodal Preoperative Localization Improves Outcomes in Reoperative Parathyroidectomy: A 25-Year Surgical Experience. *Am. Surg.* **2019**, *85*, 939–943. [CrossRef] [PubMed]
14. Philippon, M.; Guerin, C.; Taïeb, D.; Vaillant, J.; Morange, I.; Brue, T.; Conte-Devolx, B.; Henry, J.-F.; Slotema, E.; Sebag, F.; et al. Bilateral neck exploration in patients with primary hyperparathyroidism and discordant imaging results: A single-centre study. *Eur. J. Endocrinol.* **2014**, *170*, 719–725. [CrossRef]
15. Langusch, C.C.; Norlen, O.; Titmuss, A.; Donoghue, K.; Holland, A.J.; Shun, A.; Delbridge, L. Focused image-guided parathyroidectomy in the current management of primary hyperparathyroidism. *Arch. Dis. Child.* **2015**, *100*, 924–927. [CrossRef]
16. Ilgan, S.; Ozbas, S.; Bilezikci, B.; Sengezer, T.; Aydin, O.U.; Gursoy, A.; Kocak, S. Radioguided occult lesion localization for minimally invasive parathyroidectomy: Technical consideration and feasibility. *Nucl. Med. Commun.* **2014**, *35*, 1167–1174. [CrossRef]
17. Wade, T.J.; Yen, T.W.F.; Amin, A.L.; Evans, D.B.; Wilson, S.D.; Wang, T.S. Focused parathyroidectomy with intraoperative parathyroid hormone monitoring in patients with lithium-associated primary hyperparathyroidism. *Surgery* **2013**, *153*, 718–722. [CrossRef]
18. Yavuz, S.; Simonds, W.F.; Weinstein, L.S.; Collins, M.T.; Kebebew, E.; Nilubol, N.; Phan, G.Q.; Libutti, S.K.; Remaley, A.T.; Van Deventer, M.; et al. Sleeping parathyroid tumor: Rapid hyperfunction after removal of the dominant tumor. *J. Clin. Endocrinol. Metab.* **2012**, *97*, 1834–1841. [CrossRef] [PubMed]
19. Buła, G.; Truchanowski, W.; Koziołek, H.; Polczyk, J.; Ziora, P.; Gawrychowski, J. A follow-up study of patients with MEN syndromes—Five case reports. *Endokrynol. Pol.* **2018**, *69*, 163–167. [CrossRef] [PubMed]
20. Nicholson, K.J.; McCoy, K.L.; Witchel, S.F.; Stang, M.T.; Carty, S.E.; Yip, L. Comparative characteristics of primary hyperparathyroidism in pediatric and young adult patients. *Surgery* **2016**, *160*, 1008–1016. [CrossRef]
21. Flynn, M.B.; Quayyum, M.; Goldstein, R.E.; Bumpous, J.M. Outpatient parathyroid surgery: Ten-year experience: Is it safe? *Am Surg.* **2015**, *81*, 472–477. [CrossRef]
22. Schneider, D.F.; Mazeh, H.; Sippel, R.S.; Chen, H. Is minimally invasive parathyroidectomy associated with greater recurrence compared to bilateral exploration? Analysis of more than 1000 cases. *Surgery* **2012**, *152*, 1008–1015. [CrossRef]

23. Witteveen, J.E.; Van Thiel, S.; Romijn, J.A.; Hamdy, N.A.T. Therapy of endocrine disease: Hungry bone syndrome: Still a challenge in the post-operative management of primary hyperparathyroidism: A systematic review of the literature. *Eur. J. Endocrinol.* **2013**, *168*, R45–R53. [CrossRef]
24. Tachibana, S.; Sato, S.; Yokoi, T.; Nagaishi, R.; Akehi, Y.; Yanase, T.; Yamashita, H. Severe hypocalcemia complicated by postsurgical hypoparathyroidism and hungry bone syndrome in a patient with primary hyperparathyroidism, Graves' disease, and acromegaly. *Intern. Med.* **2012**, *51*, 1869–1873. [CrossRef]
25. Seib, C.D.; Chomsky-Higgins, K.; Gosnell, J.E.; Shen, W.T.; Suh, I.; Duh, Q.-Y.; Finlayson, E. Patient Frailty Should Be Used to Individualize Treatment Decisions in Primary Hyperparathyroidism. *World J. Surg.* **2018**, *42*, 3215–3222. [CrossRef]
26. Jannasch, O.; Voigt, C.; Reschke, K.; Lippert, H.; Mroczkowski, P. Comparison of Outcome Between Older and Younger Patients Following Surgery for Primary Hyperparathyroidism. *Pol. J. Surg.* **2013**, *85*, 598–604. [CrossRef]
27. Cinamon, U.; Gavish, D.; Tamir, S.O.; Goldfarb, A.; Ezri, T. Effect of general anesthesia and intubation on parathyroid levels in normal patients and those with hyperparathyroidism. *Head Neck* **2017**, *40*, 555–560. [CrossRef] [PubMed]
28. Riss, P.; Krall, C.; Scheuba, C.; Bieglmayer, C.; Niederle, B. Risk factors for "PTH spikes" during surgery for primary hyperparathyroidism. *Langenbeck's Arch. Surg.* **2013**, *398*, 881–886. [CrossRef] [PubMed]
29. Egan, R.J.; Dewi, F.; Arkell, R.; Ansell, J.; Zouwail, S.; Scott-Coombes, D.; Stechman, M. Does elective parathyroidectomy for primary hyperparathyroidism affect renal function? A prospective cohort study. *Int. J. Surg.* **2016**, *27*, 138–141. [CrossRef] [PubMed]
30. Kluijfhout, W.P.; Beninato, T.; Drake, F.T.; Vriens, M.R.; Gosnell, J.; Shen, W.T.; Suh, I.; Liu, C.; Duh, Q.Y. Unilateral Clearance for Primary Hyperparathyroidism in Selected Patients with Multiple Endocrine Neoplasia Type 1. *World J. Surg.* **2016**, *40*, 2964–2969. [CrossRef]
31. Norlén, O.; Wang, K.C.; Tay, Y.K.; Johnson, W.R.; Grodski, S.; Yeung, M.; Serpell, J.; Sidhu, S.; Sywak, M.; Delbridge, L. No Need to Abandon Focused Parathyroidectomy. *Ann. Surg.* **2015**, *261*, 991–996. [CrossRef]
32. Liu, C.; Wu, B.; Huang, P.; Ding, Q.; Xiao, L.; Zhang, M.; Zhou, J. US-Guided Percutaneous Microwave Ablation for Primary Hyperparathyroidism with Parathyroid Nodules: Feasibility and Safety Study. *J. Vasc. Interv. Radiol.* **2016**, *27*, 867–875. [CrossRef] [PubMed]
33. Lou, I.; Balentine, C.; Clarkson, S.; Schneider, D.F.; Sippel, R.S.; Chen, H. How long should we follow patients after apparently curative parathyroidectomy? *Surgery* **2017**, *161*, 54–61. [CrossRef] [PubMed]
34. Lai, V.; Yen, T.W.F.; Doffek, K.; Carr, A.A.; Carroll, T.B.; Fareau, G.G.; Evans, U.B.; Wang, T.S. Delayed Calcium Normalization After Presumed Curative Parathyroidectomy is Not Associated with the Development of Persistent or Recurrent Primary Hyperparathyroidism. *Ann. Surg. Oncol.* **2016**, *23*, 2310–2314. [CrossRef] [PubMed]

Publisher's Note: MDPI stays neutral with regard to jurisdictional claims in published maps and institutional affiliations.

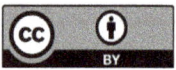

© 2020 by the authors. Licensee MDPI, Basel, Switzerland. This article is an open access article distributed under the terms and conditions of the Creative Commons Attribution (CC BY) license (http://creativecommons.org/licenses/by/4.0/).

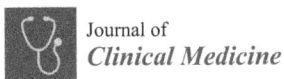

Article

Snail-1 Overexpression Correlates with Metastatic Phenotype in BRAF^{V600E} Positive Papillary Thyroid Carcinoma

Katarzyna Wieczorek-Szukala [1], Janusz Kopczynski [2], Aldona Kowalska [3,4] and Andrzej Lewinski [1,*]

[1] Department of Endocrinology and Metabolic Diseases, Medical University of Lodz, 93-338 Lodz, Poland; katarzyna.wieczorek@umed.lodz.pl
[2] Department of Pathology, Holy Cross Cancer Center, 25-734 Kielce, Poland; janusz.kopczynski@onkol.kielce.pl
[3] Endocrinology Clinic, Holy Cross Cancer Center, 25-734 Kielce, Poland; aldona.kowalska@onkol.kielce.pl
[4] Faculty of Medicine and Health Sciences, Jan Kochanowski University, 25-319 Kielce, Poland
[*] Correspondence: andrzej.lewinski@umed.lodz.pl; Tel.: +48-42-271-11-41; Fax: +48-42-271-11-40

Received: 24 July 2020; Accepted: 18 August 2020; Published: 21 August 2020

Abstract: The ability of cancer to metastasize is regulated by various signaling pathways, including transforming growth factor β (TGFβ), also implicated in the upregulation of Snail-1 transcription factor in malignant neoplasms. B-type Raf kinase gene (BRAF)^{V600E}, the most common driving mutation in papillary thyroid carcinoma (PTC), induces epithelial to mesenchymal transition (EMT) in thyroid cancer cells through changes in the Snail-1 level, increasing cell migration and invasion. However, little is known about the mechanism of Snail-1 and BRAF^{V600E} relations in humans. Our study included 61 PTC patients with evaluated BRAF^{V600E} mutation status. A total of 18 of those patients had lymph node metastases—of whom 10 were BRAF^{V600E} positive, and 8 negative. Our findings indicate that the expression of Snail-1, but not TGFβ1, correlates with the metastatic phenotype in PTC. This is the first piece of evidence that the upregulation of Snail-1 corresponds with the presence of BRAF^{V600E} mutation and increased expression of Snail-1 in metastatic PTC samples is dependent on BRAF^{V600E} mutation status.

Keywords: PTC; thyroid; metastasis; Snail-1; BRAF^{V600E}

1. Introduction

Papillary thyroid carcinoma (PTC) is the most common thyroid cancer accounting for 80–85% of all thyroid cancer cases. Although its incidence is gradually growing, the cancer-related mortality rate is relatively stable, and PTC has a good prognosis with an average 5-year survival rate of above 90% [1]. However, above 50% of PTC case often have performed local lymph node metastasis and approximately 10% of PTC cases represent aggressive metastatic neoplasm with distant metastases to lungs or bones [2]. In addition to an increased rate of primary tumors, there has been also growing incidence of regional and distant PTC metastases, which obviously increases the global need for improving our understanding of pathogenesis process and identifying effective, targeted treatments.

The fundamental mechanism by which epithelial-derived tumor cells may become malignant and obtain an invasive phenotype is the epithelial to mesenchymal transition (EMT). EMT is essential to both physiological developmental processes, as well as metastatic cancer. Numerous studies have demonstrated that this process is aberrantly activated during thyroid cancer development [3,4]. Moreover, it was discovered both in vitro and in vivo that thyroid tumour cells from PTCs and anaplastic cancer (ATCs) may constitutively display an active EMT process when compared to normal thyrocytes. This results in the loss of cells' polarity, decreased expression of particular epithelial markers and increased expression of mesenchymal markers [5,6].

It is currently known that EMT may be initialized and maintained by various molecular factors, including an inflammatory cytokine-transformation growth factor-β (TGF-β) [3]. Transforming growth factor β (TGFβ) is one of the most abundant cytokines that regulates many biological processes such as cell differentiation, apoptosis, proliferation, and other physiological and pathological conditions. TGFβ1 is thought to be the primary isoform which is overexpressed in many tumor types and may promote tumor invasion and metastasis through multiple Smad-independent or non-canonical signaling pathways [7,8]. The TGFβ family of signaling molecules has been implicated in the upregulation of key transcription factors such as Twist, Zeb or Snail-1 [8,9]. Importantly, it has been also discovered that such transcription factors may initiate the EMT process itself [3,10].

Snail-1 belongs to a family of zinc-finger transcription factors and its primary function is the repression of E-cadherin, which results in reduced cell adhesion and promotes migratory capacity [9,11]. In addition, Snail-1 activation induces fibrosis in various organs such as the kidneys, liver and lungs. The pathological activation of Snail-1 probably contributes to organ fibrosis which may further lead to chronic inflammation and cancer [12]. Snail-1 has been also recently implicated in the regulation of drug resistance and the induction of the cancer stem cell (CSC) phenotype [9,13].

However, the induction of the EMT process in the context of cancer invasion remains Snail-1's most studied function. A large number of studies have found that metastatic tumors of the colon, breast, ovary and prostate carcinomas overexpress the Snail-1 protein [9,14]. Its overexpression is generally correlated with aggressiveness, lymph node metastases (LNM), tumor recurrence and poor prognosis [15,16]. Our previous experiments concerning colon adenocarcinoma HT29 cells also indicated that Snail-1 overexpression reduced cell adhesion and increased migratory properties, which coincides with the above observations [17]. Furthermore, it was shown that Snail-1 may also play a key role in cancer cell cytoskeleton reorganization, while a positive correlation between Snail-1 presence and Tubulin–β3, (TUBB3) (one of the main proteins building microtubules, a major component of the eukaryotic cytoskeleton) upregulation in adenocarcinoma cell lines has been observed [18]. Although Snail-1 is not expressed in normal thyroid tissue, it was described to be overexpressed in different thyroid cancer cell lines [19].

PTC oncogenesis is associated with the occurrence of the mutations within the B-type Raf kinase gene–BRAF [20]. Although numerous different variants of BRAF mutations have been discovered so far, over 90% are the BRAF^{V600E} mutation. This genetic aberration influences and constantly activates the mitogen-activated protein kinase (MAPK) signaling pathway and leads to uncontrolled cell proliferation and differentiation [21]. Among other genetic alternations involving the MAPK pathway (such as RET/PTC or RAS) BRAF^{V600E} is present in more than 50% of PTC, but is rare in follicular variants, and not found in follicular thyroid cancer. Therefore, BRAF^{V600E} has been postulated as a good prognostic marker to assist in risk stratification for patients with PTC [22].

The tumorigenic role of BRAF^{V600E} in PTC development was well documented before in BRAF^{V600E} transgenic mice models. Studies performed on rat thyroid cells overexpressing BRAF^{V600E} suggested that BRAF^{V600E} is an initiator of tumorigenesis and is required for tumor progression in PTC [23]. A large number of clinical studies have demonstrated an association of BRAF^{V600E} mutation with aggressive clinicopathologic characteristics and high tumor recurrence, although the results are controversial [24].What is important, it has also been shown that BRAF^{V600E} plays a crucial role in direct EMT induction. Baquero et al. have studied this phenomenon in thyroid cancer cells and reported that BRAF^{V600E} induces EMT through changes in Snail-1 and E-cadherin protein expression levels, which in turn, increase cell migration and invasion [25]. The interaction of BRAF^{V600E} and Snail-1 has been observed also in other cancer types. Interestingly, Massoumi et al. have reported that hyperactivation of the BRAF^{V600E} mutant in melanoma cells resulted in Snail-1 overexpression and increased their metastatic potential. Introducing mutated BRAF into primary melanocytes led to increased Snail-1 expression after malignant transformation, constitutively high ERK activity and resulted in acquisition of a more aggressive cell phenotype [26].

An association has been suggested between BRAF^{V600E} and TGFβ in aggressiveness induction of PTCs. It has been shown in rat thyroid cells overexpressing BRAF^{V600E} that this oncogene stimulates TGFβ secretion, and both proteins exert the same effect on both E-cadherin expression and cell invasion [27]. However, the above studies, based on animal or cell line models (mostly anaplastic thyroid cancer model), may not fully represent the interactions between Snail-1 and BRAF^{V600E} mutation in PTC in vivo.

The aim of our study was to determine whether there is any correlation between *Snail-1* and *TGFβ1* gene expression and the existence of BRAF^{V600E} mutation in patients with metastatic or non-metastatic PTC. To our knowledge, this study is the first attempt assessing the expression of the above EMT markers and the metastatic potential of PTC in paraffin slides containing human PTC collected during surgery.

2. Materials and Methods

2.1. Patients

The study group was recruited from PTC patients diagnosed and recruited to the trial during routine follow-up from 2012 at the Endocrinology Clinic of the Holy Cross Cancer Center (Kielce, Poland). Thin-section paraffin-embedded slides of thyroid tissues were prepared by a Holycross Cancer Centre pathologist at the time of diagnosis as decribed earlier [28,29]. One of our pathologists (J. K.) marked the area containing primary tumour foci on one haematoxylin and eosin-stained slide (red line, Figure 1).

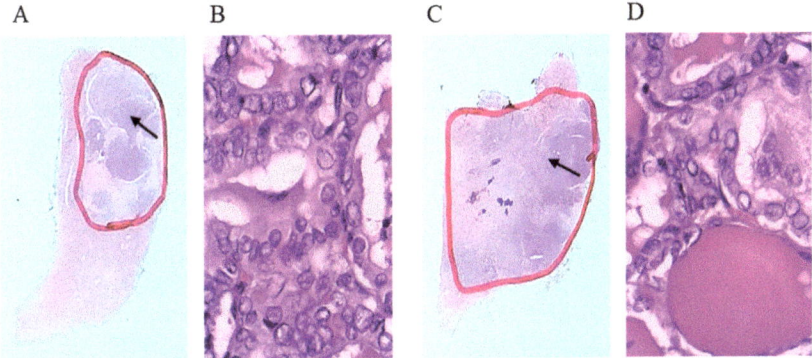

Figure 1. Representative cancer foci images. Hematoxylin and eosin staining of 2 different papillary thyroid carcinoma (PTC) samples-the primary tumour foci have been marked by pathologist (red line) (**A**,**C**). The images (**B**,**D**) show magnification ×400.

A total of 61 PTC specimens were chosen for further analysis. All the study procedures were approved by the Bioethical Committee at the Holy Cross Medical Chamber, Kielce (no. 2/2013). Patients provided their written consent for molecular tests. The patient characteristics are described in Table 1.

The presence of the V600E mutation in the BRAF gene was evaluated by three genotyping methods: allele-specific amplification PCR (ASA-PCR), qPCR, and Seq as described previously by Kowalik et al. [29]. Within the 61 patients in this study, 30 samples were BRAF^{V600E} positive and 31 BRAF^{V600E} negative. Within 18 patients with lymph node metastasis–10 were BRAF^{V600E} positive, and 8 negative. Controls were obtained from surrounding normal tissue after pathologist supervision.

Table 1. Characteristics of papillary thyroid cancer patients from whom PTC tissue has been collected.

Characteristics	n	%
Sex		
Male	10	16.4
Female	51	83.6
Age (years)		
>55	13	39.3
≤55	48	60.7
T classification		
T1–T2	26	42.6
T3–T4	35	57.4
Lymph Node Metastasis		
positive	18	29.5
negative	43	70.5
Distant Metastasis		
positive	3	4.9
negative	58	95.1
$BRAF^{V600E}$ mutation		
positive	30	49
negative	31	51

2.2. Molecular Methods

The pathologist marked the area containing PTC tumor cells on a hematoxylin and eosin-stained slide. Then, 4 to 5 unstained slides were deparaffinized by soaking twice in xylene for 15 min, twice in 96% alcohol for 5 min and once in distilled water. Tissue was scraped from thepathologist-selected area with a scalpel and transferred to a test tube for further RNA isolation.

RNA isolation has been performed using a High Pure FFPE RNA Isolation Kit (Roche, Switzerland), according to the manufacturer's protocol. The purity and integrity of total RNA was assessed by an Agilent 2100 Bioanalyzer. The degradation rate of total RNA was determined using RIN values. Only the samples with RIN > 7 were further analyzed. Total RNA was used in the first strand cDNA synthesis with a Maxima First Strand cDNA Synthesis Kit for RT-qPCR with dsDNase (Thermo Scientific, Waltham, MA, USA) according to manufacturer's instructions. RT-qPCR was performed on the ABI PRISM® 7500 Sequence Detection System (Applied Biosystem, CA, USA) by using TaqMan Gene Expression Assays and TaqMan™ Fast Advanced Master Mix according to the manufacturer's specification. The Assays Identification numbers were: SNAI1-Hs00195591_m1; TGFβ1-Hs00998133_m1; GAPDH Hs99999905_m1. Thermal cycler conditions were as follows: 2 min at 50 °C, hold for 20 s at 95 °C, followed by two-step PCR for 40 cycles of 95 °C for 3 s followed by 60 °C for 30 s. Amplification reactions, in triplicate for each sample, were performed and the results were normalized to the GAPDH gene expression level. An analysis of relative gene expression data was performed, using the 2–ΔΔCT method. The calibrator was prepared as mean gene expression values for normal tissue from 12 patients.

2.3. Statistics

The statistical analysis was carried out using the Statistica 12 software (StatsoftPolska, Kraków, Poland). A graphical representation of the results was prepared using the SigmaPlot 11 software (Systat Software Inc., San Jose, CA, USA). The results are presented as the mean of three independent experiments ± SD. The normality of the distribution was assessed using the Shapiro–Wilk test. The Student's *t*-test was used for normally distributed parameters. Chi-square tests and *t*-test were used in the medical history analysis. In all the analyses, results were considered statistically significant when $p < 0.05$.

3. Results

3.1. Snail-1, but not TGFβ1 Expression is Correlated with Metastatic Phenotype in PTC

The EMT process may be induced both through transcription factors such as Snail-1 or growth factor TGFβ1. Altered expression of those genes has been observed previously in thyroid cancer cell line models [4,25]. We analyzed the expression of those two genes in 61 FFPE tissues from PTC patients. A total of 18 PTC samples were representing metastases (18 lymph node, with three distant—as described in Table 1)—described later as "Metastatic PTC", and 43 PTC samples had no diagnosed metastases ("Non-metastatic PTC"). RT-qPCR was performed using TaqMan Gene Expression Assays. We observed a statistically significant ($p < 0.001$), more than 2.5-fold increase in *Snail-1* gene expression in metastatic PTC samples as compared to non-metastatic samples (Figure 2, grey bars). The expression of the *TGFβ1* gene in non-metastatic PTC patients was slightly higher, however, no statistical significance for this tendency between the studied groups was noted.

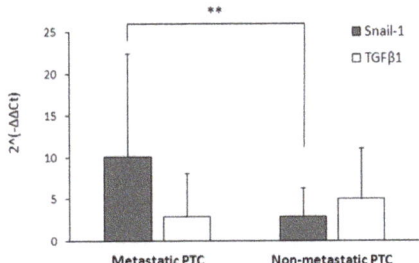

Figure 2. The expression of *Snail-1* but not *TGFβ1* was correlated with the metastatic phenotype in PTC samples. The gene expression was evaluated by quantitative RT-qPCR in metastatic ($n = 18$) and non-metastatic ($n = 43$) PTC groups. The relative mRNA level was normalized to GAPDH. The results are presented as the mean of three independent experiments ± SD. ** $p < 0.001$.

3.2. The Presence of BRAF^{V600E} Mutation Associates with Snail-1 Expression in PTC

As described before, Snail-1 protein expression may be regulated by BRAF^{V600E} mutation in human thyroid cancer cells [25]. Therefore, we divided our studied group into BRAF^{V600E} positive (30 patients) and BRAF^{V600E} negative samples (31 patients). The presence of the V600E mutation in BRAF gene was evaluated previously [14]. *Snail-1* mRNA expression was significantly higher (ca. 2-fold) in PTC with BRAF^{V600E} mutation in comparison to BRAF^{V600E} negative samples ($p < 0.05$) (Figure 3). However, the expression *TGFβ1* did not differ between those two groups.

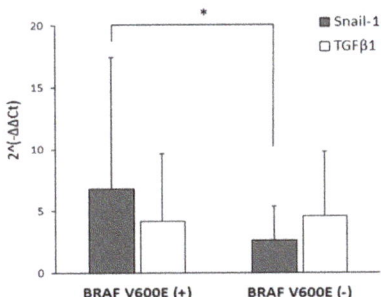

Figure 3. The expression of *Snail-1* is correlated with the presence of B-type Raf kinase gene (BRAF)^{V600E} mutation in PTC samples. The gene expression was evaluated by quantitative RT-qPCR in BRAFV600E (+) ($n = 30$) and BRAFV600E (−) ($n = 31$) PTC groups. The relative mRNA level was normalized to GAPDH. The results are presented as the mean of three independent experiments ± SD. * $p < 0.05$.

3.3. The Upregulation of Snail-1 in Metastatic PTC Samples is Dependent on BRAF^{V600E} Mutation Status

Furthermore, we aimed to evaluate the role of BRAF^{V600E} mutation on the expression of *Snail-1* and *TGFβ1* within metastatic PTC samples. Among 18 PTC patients with lymph node metastasis–10 samples harboured BRAF^{V600E} mutation (described later as "Metastatic- BRAF V600E (+)"), and 8 were BRAFV600E negative ("Metastatic–BRAF V600E (−)"). Among 43 PTC patients with no diagnosed metastases—20 were BRAF^{V600E} positive ("Non-metastatic–BRAF V600E (+)"), and 23 BRAF^{V600E} negative ("Non-metastatic–BRAF V600E (−)").

Snail-1 expression level was nearly 3-fold higher in metastatic PTC that harbored the BRAF^{V600E} mutation when compared to the metastatic but BRAF^{V600E} negative group ($p < 0.05$) (Figure 4A, grey bars). Interestingly, the expression level of the *Snail-1* gene in metastatic but BRAF^{V600E} negative PTC samples (Figure 4A) remained on a similar level as in the non-metastatic PTC patients, regardless of BRAF^{V600E} mutation status (Figure 4B).

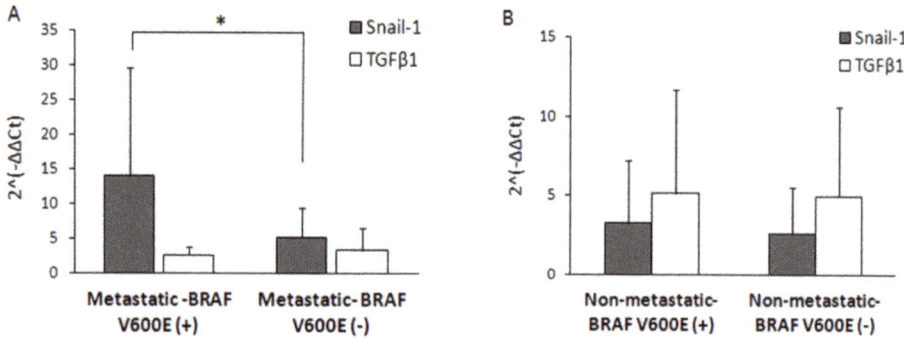

Figure 4. The upregulation of *Snail-1* in metastatic PTC samples is dependent on BRAF^{V600E} mutation status. The gene expression was evaluated by quantitative RT-qPCR in both BRAF V600E (+) ($n = 10$) and BRAF V600E (−) metastatic ($n = 8$) (**A**) and non-metastatic BRAF V600E (+) ($n = 20$) and BRAF V600E (−) ($n = 23$) PTC groups (**B**). The relative mRNA level was normalized to GAPDH. The results are presented as the mean of three independent experiments ± SD. * $p < 0.05$.

On the other hand, in both metastatic and non-metastatic PTC groups: BRAF V600E (+) or (−) (Figure 4A,B, white bars), no significant differences in *TGFβ1* gene expression levels were found (Student's *t*-test, $p > 0.05$ in each case).

Table 2 summarizes some vital clinical features of the studied metastatic and non-metastatic PTC patient groups. Statistical analysis showed no significant statistical correlation between BRAF^{V600E} mutation status in PTC tissue and gender, age at diagnosis, or T-classification of the primary tumor. However, it was observed that significantly more samples of non-metastatic PTC tumors with T3–T4 classification harbored the BRAF^{V600E} mutation. Furthermore, it can be observed that more patients with non-metastatic and BRAF^{V600E} negative PTC had been diagnosed as less advanced T1–T2 tumor stage ($p = 0.0002$). Nevertheless, due to the limited number of patients in the studied groups evaluation of such analysis requires further research.

Table 2. Clinical features of metastatic and non-metastatic PTC tumors with or without BRAF^{V600E} mutation, ** $p < 0.001$.

Clinical Features	Metastatic Tumors			Non-Metastatic Tumors		
	BRAF^{V600E} Positive ($n = 10$)	BRAF^{V600E} Negative ($n = 8$)	p-Value	BRAF^{V600E} Positive ($n = 20$)	BRAF^{V600E} Negative ($n = 23$)	p-Value
Gender						
Male	4/10 (40%)	1/8 (12.5%)	0.120	2/20 (10%)	3/23 (13%)	0.400
Female	6/10 (60%)	7/8 (87.5%)		18/20 (90%)	20/23 (87%)	
Age at Diagnosis (years)						
Mean ±SD	54 ± 14	49 ± 15	0.506	55 ± 12	47 ± 15	0.050
≤55	6/10 (60%)	5/8 (62.5%)	0.501	10/20 (50%)	17/23 (74%)	0.110
>55	4/10 (40%)	3/8 (37.5%)		10/20 (50%)	6/23 (26%)	
T Classification						
T1–T2	2/10 (20%)	3/8 (37.5%)	0.200	7/20 (35%)	18/23 (78%)	0.0002 **
T3–T4	8/10 (80%)	5/8 (62.5%)		13/20 (65%)	5/23 (22%)	

4. Discussion

PTC is the most common of all thyroid cancers, with a gradually growing incidence. The majority of PTC cases generally present good prognosis with conventional therapies. Nevertheless, approximately 10% of PTC cases progress to more aggressive forms associated with local invasion, distant metastases and poorer clinical outcome [1,2]. Despite metastasis remaining the key cause of failure in cancer treatment and mortality, its molecular mechanisms remain poorly examined.

Metastatic process is associated with change of phenotype due to the epithelial–mesenchymal transition (EMT), an essential physiological mechanism in embryonic development and tissue repair. However, EMT may also contribute to the progression of disease, such as organ fibrosis or cancer [3]. This process results from the induction of transcription factors that change gene expression, therefore promoting the loss of cell–cell adhesion, modifying cytoskeletal dynamics and leading to a change from epithelial morphology and physiology to the mesenchymal phenotype. EMT can be induced by various signaling pathways, for example mediated by transforming growth factor β (TGFβ), Wnt–β-catenin, Notch, Hedgehog receptor tyrosine kinases (RTK) [4,5].

The role of TGFβ in cancer is complex: this pathway may function both in tumor suppression and in tumor promotion. TGFβ also functions as a tumor suppressor in early tumor development. In a number of human cancers, TGFβ inhibits cell cycle progression, increases apoptosis, and suppresses the expression of growth factors, cytokines, and chemokines. The function of *TGFβ* as a tumor suppressor or a tumor promoter depends on the context and stage of tumor progression. Its shift to a pro-metastatic role at later tumor stages has been shown to be mediated by various signaling pathways [7,10].

The thyroid gland expresses the *TGFβ1* gene mRNA and synthesizes the protein, which under physiologic conditions regulates thyroid growth and function. Interestingly, it was concluded that the alterations in the signaling pathway of *TGFβ1* are not the same in tumors from different species [7]. It seems it is not entirely possible to apply the results obtained in animal or cell culture studies to normal or pathological human thyroid tissue. It should be noted that using a single experimental research model usually entails some limitations. For example, employing exclusively tissue material collected from patients, may lead to a somehow less comprehensive scientific reasoning.

The studies of the expression of *TGFβ1* performed before in human PTC revealed that, when compared to the central areas, the peripheral invasive areas of the tumors had increased expression of *TGFβ1*, *NFkβ*, and CDC42 as well as showing a decrease in cell–cell adhesion proteins. Moreover, these regions presented also an overexpression of vimentin, a characteristic marker of EMT. The authors concluded that these changes might be related to increased tumor invasiveness and suggest an important role of TGFβ as inductor of EMT and metastasis [5,7]. Other studies of Brace et al. have shown that *TGFβ1*, but not *TGFβ2*, is significantly increased in PTC compared to benign thyroid nodules and therefore may serve as a potential diagnostic marker [30].

However, in our studies, no statistically significant differences were found in *TGFβ1* gene expression in BRAF V600E (+) and BRAF V600E (−) PTC groups, as well as in PTC metastatic samples with known BRAFV600E mutation status. Possibly, this may result from the fact that TGFβ has been found overexpressed locally in the invasive front of cancer cells, also in different cancer types, for example in the breast cancer [31]. Moreover, in ovarian cancer Wang et al. have demonstrated that the expression of TGF-β1 is not associated with lymphatic metastasis [32]. Moreover, it has been discovered that BRAF^{V600E} increases exclusively *TGFβ1* secretion through the MEK/ERK pathway in thyroid tumour cells [27]. The observations of Riesco-Eizaguirre et al. have led to the concept that the action of TGFβ in PTC is very important locally as a modulator of the tumor microenvironment, however, the total *TGFβ1* expression may not be altered [33].

It has been widely described that the TGFβ cascade also induces the expression of Snail-1-a zinc finger transcription factor, the main E-cadherin repressor and one of the most potent EMT inducers [34]. Snail-1 was found to be overexpressed in the invasive fronts of several human tumors derived from epithelial cells [4,14] and proved to play a key role in PTC, as well. Although Snail-1 is not expressed in normal thyroid tissue, histopathological analyses have proved that the expression of Snail-1 protein was mainly located in the cytoplasm and nuclei of PTC cells [19]. The overexpression of this gene and the upregulated protein level have been discovered in numerous cancer types such as ovarian and breast carcinomas, melanomas, oral squamous carcinomas, human thyroid carcinomas and their metastases. In the context of thyroid cancers, the effects of Snail-1 interactions have not been thoroughly studied or understood. It has been suggested that Snail-1 expression, together with TGFβ1, is associated with lymph node metastasis in PTC and may be a potential biomarker of tumor diagnosis and prognosis in PTC [8].

Interestingly, Baquero et al. have discovered that Snail-1 expression may also be regulated by BRAF^{V600E}—the most common mutation found in PTCs [25]. In the thyroid carcinoma cell model, BRAF^{V600E} induced EMT via changes in Snail-1 and E-cadherin protein expression levels, which in turn increased the migration and invasiveness of these cells. Moreover, inhibition of BRAF^{V600E} significantly decreased invasion of thyroid cancer cells, tumor volume and metastases in a mouse model of anaplastic thyroid carcinoma [25,27].

In our studies, it was observed that BRAF^{V600E} mutation was present in significantly more cases of non-metastatic aggressive tumors (with T3–T4 classification). However, due to the limited number of patients in the studied groups, such statistics should be evaluated with some perspective.

Most clinical research has demonstrated an association between BRAF^{V600E} mutation status, aggressive clinicopathologic characteristics of PTC and high tumor recurrence, although the results remain controversial [24]. Contradictory results from other groups have stressed that, although BRAF^{V600E} mutation may show very high prevalence of the *BRAF* mutation in PTC in the population, the presence of the mutation itself was not statistically associated with a metastasis, patient age, completeness of resection, local invasion or tumor size score. Although BRAF^{V600E} analysis may have some value in distinguishing malignant and benign thyroid tumors, it is currently believed that alone it is not a good predictor of more the aggressive clinical course of PTC [28].

Therefore, we have aimed to evaluate if *Snail-1* and *TGFβ1* genes expression correlate with one another in human PTC tissue samples or whether they are related to BRAF^{V600E} mutation status or LNM tumor staging. We demonstrate that *Snail-1* gene expression is significantly increased in metastatic PTC patients group (based on LNM scale) in comparison to non-metastatic samples. Moreover, we show that *Snail-1* elevated expression also correlates with BRAF^{V600E} positive status. Our results clearly correspond with the data obtained by Baquero et al. on the cellular model [25]. On the contrary, Mitchell et al., utilizing immunohistochemical techniques, suggested that Snail-1 protein expression did not correlate with BRAF status and E-cadherin expression in PTC [35]. Such discrepancies may result from different molecular techniques, or the relatively small number of studied patient samples. It must be also emphasized that Snail-1 protein is relatively unstable, and in the cytoplasm, it may be prone to proteasomal degradation, with a half-life of only twenty-five minutes. GSK3β is a Snail kinase can bind to and phosphorylate this transcription factor, facilitating its degradation. Phosphorylation determines Snail-1's subcellular location, as GSK-3β-mediated phosphorylation induces Snail-1 export to the cytoplasm [9,36]. Therefore, every study concerning Snail-1 protein expression should also consider its localization.

Interestingly, for the first time using human PTC tissue model, our findings reveal that *Snail-1* gene expression was significantly higher exclusively in metastatic PTC that harbored the BRAF^{V600E} mutation, but not in metastatic BRAF^{V600E}-negative PTC tissue. In contrast, we did not observe such differences in *Snail-1* gene expression in non-metastatic PTC patients, regardless of BRAF^{V600E} mutation status. This may suggest that in cells altered by metastatic processes, such as EMT, BRAF^{V600E} mutation facilitates the mechanism of *Snail-1* overexpression. It has previously been proposed that BRAF^{V600E} can increase Snail-1 expression both at transcriptional level and via GSK3β inhibition [27]. However, the mechanism of transcription regulation in the presence of BRAF mutation remains to be further elucidated.

Despite some limitations of our study resulting from the relatively small sample size due to the selection of metastasizing PTC cases, caused by only one mutation of individual gene (BRAF^{V600E}), the presented data confirm that BRAF^{V600E} participates in mechanisms involved in the increase in *Snail-1* expression in metastatic PTC. Possibly, the interplay between BRAF^{V600E} and *Snail-1* may play a key role in the thyroid gland neoplastic transformation and cancer cell invasiveness. The further elucidation of the mutual interactions between *Snail-1* and BRAF^{V600E} mutation in PTC in vivo may shed new light on the issue of metastatic thyroid cancer development. Better understanding of its complexity would help to identify specific targets for modern molecular therapies and develop more accurate diagnostic strategies.

Author Contributions: Conceptualization, K.W.-S. and A.L.; methodology, K.W.-S. and J.K.; resources, A.K.; writing—original draft preparation, K.W.-S.; writing—review and editing, A.L.; supervision, A.L. All authors have read and agreed to the published version of the manuscript.

Funding: This study was financially supported by the Medical University of Lodz, project No 502-03/1-107-03/502-14-316 and statutory funds 503/1-107-03/503-11-001-19-00.

Conflicts of Interest: The authors declare no conflict of interest.

Abbreviations

PTC	Papillary thyroid carcinoma
AT	Anaplastic thyroid carcinoma
EMT	Epithelial to mesenchymal transition
TGF	Transformation growth factor
CSC	Cancer stem cells
LNM	Lymph node metastases
MAPK	Mitogen-activated protein kinase
TUBB3	Tubulin –β3, RTK-Receptor tyrosine kinases

References

1. Agrawal, N.; Akbani, R.; Aksoy, B.A.; Ally, A.; Arachchi, H.; Asa, S.L.; Auman, J.T.; Balasundaram, M.; Balu, S.; Baylin, S.B.; et al. Integrated Genomic Characterization of Papillary Thyroid Carcinoma. *Cell* **2014**, *159*, 676–690. [CrossRef] [PubMed]
2. Schlumberger, M.; Pacini, F.; Tuttle, R.M. *Thyroid Tumors*, 3rd ed.; Estimprim: Autechaux, France, 2015; pp. 221–234.
3. Coghlin, C.; Murray, G. Current and emerging concepts in tumour metastasis. *J. Pathol.* **2010**, *222*, 1–15. [CrossRef] [PubMed]
4. Tania, M.; Khan, M.A.; Fu, J. Epithelial to mesenchymal transition inducing transcription factors and metastatic cancer. *Tumor Biol.* **2014**, *35*, 7335–7342. [CrossRef] [PubMed]

5. Shakib, H.; Rajabi, S.; Dehghan, M.; Mashayekhi, F.J.; Safari-Alighiarloo, N.; Hedayati, M. Epithelial-to-mesenchymal transition in thyroid cancer: A comprehensive review. *Endocrine* **2019**, *66*, 435–455. [CrossRef]
6. Liu, Z.; Kakudo, K.; Bai, Y.; Li, Y.; Ozaki, T.; Miyauchi, A.; Taniguchi, E.; Mori, I. Loss of cellular polarity/cohesiveness in the invasive front of papillary thyroid carcinoma, a novel predictor for lymph node metastasis; possible morphological indicator of epithelial mesenchymal transition. *J. Clin. Pathol.* **2011**, *64*, 325–329. [CrossRef] [PubMed]
7. Pisarev, M.A.; Thomasz, L.; Juvenal, G. Role of transforming growth factor beta in the regulation of thyroid function and growth. *Thyroid* **2009**, *19*, 881–892. [CrossRef] [PubMed]
8. Wang, N.; Jiang, R.; Yang, J.Y.; Tang, C.; Yang, L.; Xu, M.; Jiang, Q.F.; Liu, Z.M. Expression of TGF-β1, SNAI1 and MMP-9 is associated with lymph node metastasis in papillary thyroid carcinoma. *J. Mol. Hist.* **2014**, *45*, 391–399. [CrossRef]
9. Kaufhold, S.; Bonavida, B. Central role of Snail1 in the regulation of EMT and resistance in cancer: A target for therapeutic intervention. *J. Exp. Clin. Cancer Res.* **2014**, *33*, 62. [CrossRef]
10. Skovierova, H.; Okajcekova, T.; Strnadel, J.; Vidomanova, E.; Halasova, E. Molecular regulation of epithelial-to-mesenchymal transition in tumorigenesis. *Int. J. Mol. Med.* **2018**, *41*, 1187–1200.
11. Murray, S.A.; Gridley, T. Snail1 gene function during early embryo patterning in mice. *Cell Cycle* **2006**, *5*, 2566–2570. [CrossRef]
12. Wawro, M.E.; Sobierajska, K.; Ciszewski, W.M.; Wagner, W.; Frontczak, M.; Wieczorek, K.; Niewiarowska, J. Tubulin beta 3 and 4 are involved in the generation of early fibrotic stages. *Cell Signal.* **2017**, *38*, 26–38. [CrossRef] [PubMed]
13. Ota, I.; Masui, T.; Kurihara, M.; Yook, J.; Mikami, S.; Kimura, T.; Shimada, K.; Konishi, N.; Yane, K.; Yamanaka, T.; et al. Snail-induced EMT promotes cancer stem cell-like properties in head and neck cancer cells. *Oncol. Rep.* **2016**, *35*, 261–266. [CrossRef] [PubMed]
14. Brzozowa, M.; Michalski, M.; Wyrobiec, G.; Piecuch, A.; Dittfeld, A.; Harabin-Słowińska, M.; Boroń, D.; Wojnicz, R. The role of Snail1 transcription factor in colorectal cancer progression and metastasis. *Contemp. Oncol.* **2015**, *19*, 265–270. [CrossRef] [PubMed]
15. Shin, N.R.; Jeong, E.H.; Choi, C.; Moon, H.J.; Kwon, C.; Chu, I.S.; Kim, G.H.; Jeon, T.Y.; Kim, D.; Lee, J.; et al. Overexpression of Snail is associated with lymph node metastasis and poor prognosis in patients with gastric cancer. *BMC Cancer* **2012**, *12*, 521. [CrossRef]
16. Christofori, G. New signals from the invasive front. *Nature* **2006**, *441*, 444–450. [CrossRef]
17. Wieczorek, K.; Wiktorska, M.; Sacewicz-Hofman, I.; Boncela, J.; Lewiński, A.; Kowalska, M.A.; Niewiarowska, J. Filamin A upregulation correlates with Snail-induced epithelial to mesenchymal transition (EMT) and cell adhesion but its inhibition increases the migration of colon adenocarcinoma HT29 cells. *Exp. Cell. Res.* **2017**, *359*, 163–170. [CrossRef]
18. Sobierajska, K.; Wieczorek, K.; Ciszewski, W.M.; Sacewicz-Hofman, I.; Wawro, M.E.; Wiktorska, M.; Boncela, J.; Papiewska-Pajak, I.; Kwasniak, P.; Wyroba, E.; et al. β-III tubulin modulates the behavior of Snail overexpressed during the epithelial-to-mesenchymal transition in colon cancer cells. *J. Biochim. Biophys. Acta* **2016**, *1863*, 2221–2233. [CrossRef]
19. Yang, X.; Shi, R.; Zhang, J. Co-expression and clinical utility of Snail and N-cadherin in papillary thyroid carcinoma. *Tumor Biol.* **2016**, *37*, 413–417. [CrossRef]
20. Lewiński, A.; Adamczewski, Z.; Zygmunt, A.; Markuszewski, L.; Karbownik-Lewińska, M.; Stasiak, M. Correlations between molecular landscape and Sonographic image of different variants of papillary thyroid carcinoma. *J. Clin. Med.* **2019**, *8*, 1916. [CrossRef]
21. Tufano, R.P.; Teixeira, G.V.; Bishop, J.; Carson, K.A.; Xing, M. BRAF mutation in papillary thyroid cancer and its value in tailoring initial treatment: A systematic review and meta-analysis. *Medicine* **2012**, *91*, 274–286. [CrossRef]
22. Knauf, J.A.; Sartor, M.A.; Medvedovic, M.; Lundsmith, E.; Ryder, M.; Salzano, M.; Nikiforov, Y.E.; Giordano, T.J.; Ghossein, R.A.; Fagin, J.A. Progression of BRAF-induced thyroid cancer is associated with epithelial–mesenchymal transition requiring concomitant MAP kinase and TGF beta signaling. *Oncogene* **2011**, *30*, 3153–3162. [CrossRef] [PubMed]
23. Tang, K.; Lee, C. BRAF mutation in papillary thyroid carcinoma: Pathogenic role and clinical implications. *J. Chin. Med. Assoc.* **2010**, *73*, 113–128. [CrossRef]

24. Li, C.; Han, P.; Lee, K.C.; Lee, L.; Fox, A.C.; Beninato, T.; Thiess, M.; Dy, B.M.; Sebo, T.; Thompson, G.B.; et al. Does BRAF V600E mutation predict aggressive features in papillary thyroid cancer? Results from four endocrine surgery centers. *J. Clin. Endocrinol. Metab.* **2013**, *9*, 3702–3712. [CrossRef] [PubMed]
25. Baquero, P.; Sánchez-Hernández, I.; Jiménez-Mora, E.; Orgaz, J.L.; Jiménez, B.; Chiloeches, A. V600E BRAF promotes invasiveness of thyroid cancer cells by decreasing E-cadherin expression through a Snail-dependent mechanism. *Cancer Lett.* **2013**, *335*, 232–241. [CrossRef] [PubMed]
26. Massoumi, R.; Kuphal, S.; Hellerbrand, C.; Haas, B.; Wild, P.; Spruss, T.; Pfeifer, A.; Fässler, R.; Bosserhoff, A.K. Down-regulation of CYLD expression by Snail promotes tumor progression in malignant melanoma. *J. Exp. Med.* **2009**, *206*, 221–232. [CrossRef] [PubMed]
27. Baquero, P.; Jimenez-Mora, E.; Santos, A.; Lasa, M.; Chiloeches, A. TGFβ induces epithelial-mesenchymal transition of thyroid cancer cells by both the BRAF/MEK/ERK and Src/FAK pathways. *Mol. Carcinog.* **2016**, *55*, 1639–1654. [CrossRef]
28. Walczyk, A.; Kowalska, A.; Kowalik, A.; Sygut, J.; Wypiórkiewicz, E.; Chodurska, R.; Pięciak, L.; Góźdź, S. The BRAF (V600E) mutation in papillary thyroid microcarcinoma: Does the mutation have an impact on clinical outcome? *Clin. Endocrinol.* **2014**, *80*, 899–904. [CrossRef]
29. Kowalik, A.; Kowalska, A.; Walczyk, A.; Chodurska, R.; Kopczyński, J.; Chrapek, M.; Wypiórkiewicz, E.; Chłopek, M.; Pięciak, L.; Gąsior-Perczak, D.; et al. Evaluation of molecular diagnostic approaches for the detection of BRAF p.V600E mutations in papillary thyroid cancer: Clinical implications. *PLoS ONE* **2017**, *12*, e0179691. [CrossRef]
30. Brace, M.D.; Wang, J.; Petten, M.; Bullock, M.J.; Makki, F.; Trites, J.; Taylor, S.M.; Hart, R.D. Differential expression of transforming growth factor-beta in benign vs. papillary thyroid cancer nodules; A potential diagnostic tool? *J. Otolaryngol.-Head Neck Surg.* **2014**, *43*, 22. [CrossRef]
31. Pang, M.F.; Georgoudaki, A.M.; Lambut, L.; Johansson, J.; Tabor, V.; Hagikura, K.; Jin, Y.; Jansson, M.; Alexander, J.S.; Nelson, C.M.; et al. TGF-β1-induced EMT promotes targeted migration of breast cancer cells through the lymphatic system by the activation of CCR7/CCL21-mediated chemotaxis. *Oncogene* **2016**, *35*, 748–760. [CrossRef]
32. Wang, S.; Liu, J.; Wang, C.; Lin, B.; Hao, Y.; Wang, Y.; Gao, S.; Qi, Y.; Zhang, Y.; Iwamori, M. Expression and correlation of Lewis y antigen and TGF-β1 in ovarian epithelial carcinoma. *Oncol. Rep.* **2012**, *27*, 1065–1071. [CrossRef] [PubMed]
33. Riesco-Eizaguirre, G.; Rodríguez, I.; De la Vieja, A.; Costamagna, E.; Carrasco, N.; Nistal, M.; Santisteban, P. The BRAFV600E oncogene induces transforming growth factor β secretion leading to sodium iodide symporter repression and increased malignancy in thyroid cancer. *Cancer Res.* **2009**, *69*, 8317–8325. [CrossRef] [PubMed]
34. Dhasarathy, A.; Phadke, D.; Mav, D.; Shah, R.R.; Wade, P.A. The transcription factors Snail and Slug activate the transforming growth factor-beta signaling pathway in breast cancer. *PLoS ONE* **2011**, *6*, e26514. [CrossRef]
35. Mitchell, B.; Leone, D.A.; Feller, J.K.; Yang, S.; Mahalingam, M. BRAF and epithelial-mesenchymal transition in primary cutaneous melanoma: A role for Snail and E-cadherin? *Hum. Pathol.* **2016**, *52*, 19–27. [CrossRef] [PubMed]
36. McCubrey, J.A.; Steelman, L.S.; Bertrand, F.E.; Davis, N.M.; Sokolosky, M.; Abrams, S.L.; Montalto, G.; D'Assoro, A.B.; Libra, M.; Nicoletti, F.; et al. GSK-3 as potential target for therapeutic intervention in cancer. *Oncotarget* **2014**, *5*, 2881–2911. [CrossRef] [PubMed]

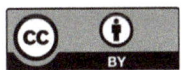

© 2020 by the authors. Licensee MDPI, Basel, Switzerland. This article is an open access article distributed under the terms and conditions of the Creative Commons Attribution (CC BY) license (http://creativecommons.org/licenses/by/4.0/).

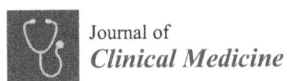

Article

S-Detect Software vs. EU-TIRADS Classification: A Dual-Center Validation of Diagnostic Performance in Differentiation of Thyroid Nodules

Ewelina Szczepanek-Parulska [1,*,†], Kosma Wolinski [1,*,†], Katarzyna Dobruch-Sobczak [2], Patrycja Antosik [1], Anna Ostalowska [1], Agnieszka Krauze [3], Bartosz Migda [3], Agnieszka Zylka [4], Malgorzata Lange-Ratajczak [5], Tomasz Banasiewicz [5], Marek Dedecjus [4], Zbigniew Adamczewski [6,7], Rafal Z. Slapa [3], Robert K. Mlosek [3], Andrzej Lewinski [6,7] and Marek Ruchala [1]

1. Department of Endocrinology, Metabolism and Internal Medicine, Poznan University of Medical Sciences, 60-355 Poznan, Poland; patrycja.antosik@gmail.com (P.A.); anna.ostalowska95@gmail.com (A.O.); mruchala@ump.edu.pl (M.R.)
2. Radiology Department II, Maria Sklodowska-Curie National Research Institute of Oncology, 02-781 Warsaw, Poland; kdsobczak@gmail.com
3. Diagnostic Imaging Department, Medical University of Warsaw, 2nd Faculty of Medicine with the English Division and the Physiotherapy Division, 03-242 Warsaw, Poland; a.kaczor@hotmail.com (A.K.); bartoszmigda@gmail.com (B.M.); rz.slapa@gmail.com (R.Z.S.); kmlosek@poczta.internetdsl.pl (R.K.M.)
4. Department of Oncological Endocrinology and Nuclear Medicine, Maria Sklodowska-Curie National Research Institute of Oncology, 02-781 Warsaw, Poland; agnieszka.zylka.edu@gmail.com (A.Z.); marek.dedecjus@gmail.com (M.D.)
5. Department of General, Endocrinological, and Oncological Surgery and Gastrointestinal Oncology, Poznan University of Medical Sciences, 60-355 Poznan, Poland; chirsk2@ump.edu.pl (M.L.-R.); tbanasie@ump.edu.pl (T.B.)
6. Department of Endocrinology and Metabolic Diseases, Medical University of Lodz, 90-419 Lodz, Poland; zbigniewadamczewski@gmail.com (Z.A.); andrzej.lewinski@office365.umed.pl (A.L.)
7. Polish Mother's Memorial Hospital-Research Institute, 93-338 Lodz, Poland
* Correspondence: ewelina@ump.edu.pl (E.S.-P.); kosma1644@poczta.onet.pl (K.W.); Tel.: +48-61-869-13-30 (E.S.-P. & K.W.)
† These authors equally contributed to this work.

Received: 11 June 2020; Accepted: 30 July 2020; Published: 3 August 2020

Abstract: Computer-aided diagnosis (CAD) and other risk stratification systems may improve ultrasound image interpretation. This prospective study aimed to compare the diagnostic performance of CAD and the European Thyroid Imaging Reporting and Data System (EU-TIRADS) classification applied by physicians with S-Detect 2 software CAD based on Korean Thyroid Imaging Reporting and Data System (K-TIRADS) and combinations of both methods (MODELs 1 to 5). In all, 133 nodules from 88 patients referred to thyroidectomy with available histopathology or with unambiguous results of cytology were included. The S-Detect system, EU-TIRADS, and mixed MODELs 1–5 for the diagnosis of thyroid cancer showed a sensitivity of 89.4%, 90.9%, 84.9%, 95.5%, 93.9%, 78.9% and 93.9%; a specificity of 80.6%, 61.2%, 88.1%, 53.7%, 73.1%, 89.6% and 80.6%; a positive predictive value of 81.9%, 69.8%, 87.5%, 67%, 77.5%, 88.1% and 82.7%; a negative predictive value of 88.5%, 87.2%, 85.5%, 92.3%, 92.5%, 81.1% and 93.1%; and an accuracy of 85%, 75.9%, 86.5%, 74.4%, 83.5%, 84.2%, and 87.2%, respectively. Comparison showed superiority of the similar MODELs 1 and 5 over other mixed models as well as EU-TIRADS and S-Detect used alone (p-value < 0.05). S-Detect software is characterized with high sensitivity and good specificity, whereas EU-TIRADS has high sensitivity, but rather low specificity. The best diagnostic performance in malignant thyroid nodule (TN) risk stratification was obtained for the combined model of S-Detect ("possibly malignant" nodule) and simultaneously obtaining 4 or 5 points (MODEL 1) or exactly 5 points (MODEL 5) on the EU-TIRADS scale.

Keywords: thyroid nodules; thyroid cancer; ultrasound; computer-aided diagnosis; S-Detect; EU-TIRADS

1. Introduction

Thyroid nodules (TNs) are the most frequent endocrine disorder and occur in 10–70% of the general population, with a relatively low malignancy rate of 3–10% [1]. The most challenging issue for medical practitioners is the differentiation between benign and malignant TNs. Ultrasonography (US) of the thyroid gland is commonly used by physicians and is crucial to decide on further management, such as qualification for fine-needle aspiration biopsy (FNAB) as well as the decision on a conservative or surgical approach [2,3]. However, the analysis of nodules' composition, echogenicity, shape, orientation, margin, calcifications, presence of halo, type of vascularization, and elasticity [4] is time consuming and subject to diverse inter-observer and intra-observer variability in the multi-ultrasound descriptor assessment of thyroid nodules, with slight to substantial agreement (κ-values ranging from 0.33 to 0.61) [5]. Moreover, no single US feature or combination of features can reliably predict the malignant character of TNs [6,7]. Furthermore, the results of US strongly depend on the operator's interpretation and experience, which implies US sensitivity and specificity varying from 52% to 81% and 54% to 83%, respectively [8,9]. In some thyroid pathologies, additional imaging methods may be applied together with US to increase its diagnostic value [10,11]. Difficulties with the interpretation of US findings often lead to redundant FNAB or even diagnostic surgery. Recently, the European Thyroid Imaging Reporting and Data System (EU-TIRADS) was established to facilitate standardization and provide a simple lexicon for distinguishing between benign and malignant TNs and to reduce the number of unnecessary invasive interventions (FNAB, thyroidectomy) [12]. A meta-analysis of seven studies, evaluating 5672 thyroid nodules, indicated that stratifying the risk of thyroid nodules by EU-TIRADS showed high performance, while the prevalence of malignancy in EU-TIRADS class 5 was equal to 76.1% [13]. Nonetheless, even this classification might be intricate for inexperienced physicians [8]. To overcome this difficulty, computer-aided diagnosis (CAD) systems are gaining interest for US image analysis and are developed on the basis of statistical data mining algorithms, collected from medical center databases. It enables non-invasive judgement on benignity or malignancy of TNs on the basis of US image analysis [14,15]. The purpose of CAD is to increase the diagnostic confidence, achieve interpretation constancy of US features, and eliminate the inter-observer variability in order to increase diagnostic accuracy, especially when the examination is performed by ultrasonographers outside referenced centers for thyroid cancer diagnostics. The practical potential of CAD has been suggested in a few recent studies [8,9,14,16]. Kwak TIRADS has high sensitivity and low specificity. Thus, it is very useful for discarding the benign cases and reducing the number of biopsies [17]. CAD is supposed to be an applicable tool in TN diagnostics and clinical decision-making for medical practitioners with basic US skills [15,16]. It may be useful especially for less experienced operators, increasing the specificity of the examination [18]. However, there is an unmet need for validation of the method on a large cohort of patients in highly referenced centers to provide reliable information on its real clinical utility and identify a target group of physicians who may benefit from the CAD-supported evaluation of TNs. Thus, the aim of our study was to compare CAD diagnostic performance with the state-of-the-art thyroid nodule classification EU-TIRADS applied by physicians based on US morphological features, in order to support decision-making regarding the further management of TNs.

2. Experimental Section

2.1. Patients

The studied group consisted of 88 patients with thyroid nodular disease. Lesions included in the study comprised nodules whose character was verified by the unambiguous diagnostic result of a fine-needle aspiration biopsy (concerning nodules presenting category II, V, or VI according to the Bethesda classification, unless the histopathological verification was performed) or nodules in patients subjected to a thyroidectomy, for whom the result of histopathological examination was available. The **exclusion criteria** for the study were as follows:

- completely cystic lesions,
- lesions with eggshell calcifications,
- lesions with indeterminate (category III or IV according to the Bethesda classification) or non-diagnostic cytology results (category I according to the Bethesda classification), if the histopathological verification was not performed.

The diagram depicting excluding factors and the process of recruitment of the patients for the study is presented in Figure 1.

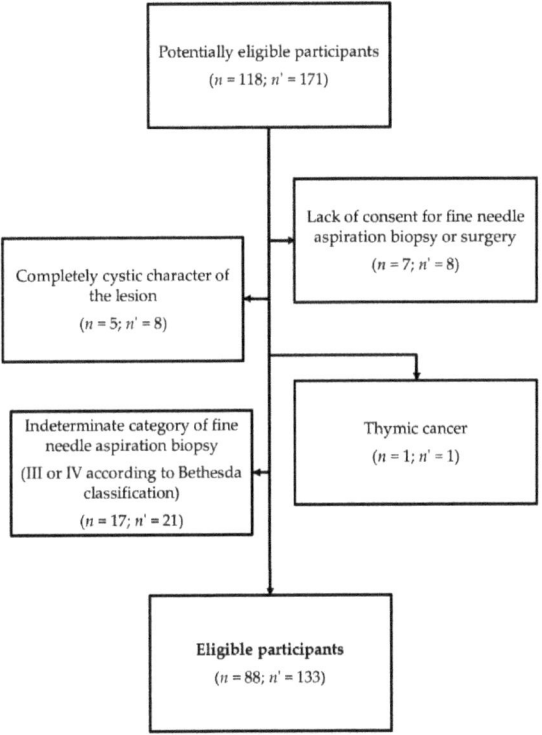

n = number of the patients

n' = number of the nodules

Figure 1. Diagram presenting the process of recruitment of the patients for the study.

2.2. Methods

This was a prospective study. Patients eligible for the study were recruited from those admitted to the tertiary reference endocrine or surgical centers for urgent evaluation of the indications for thyroidectomy due to the following results of the Bethesda System for Reporting Thyroid Cytopathology (BSRTC): (a) suspicion of malignancy or thyroid cancer (BSRTC category IV-VI or (b) nodular goiter with clinical symptoms (BSRTC category II). Nodules with category IV, V, or VI were ultimately subjected to thyroidectomy and the final result of histopathological examination served as a source of final diagnosis on the character of the lesions. In the case of patients for whom the result of the biopsy was consistent with benign lesions and who did not present with local symptoms (large goiter, compressive symptoms, dysphagia, dysphonia), they were not subjected to surgical procedure and the result of the biopsy served as the final verification of the character of the lesions.

2.2.1. Ultrasound Examination

The ultrasound examination of the thyroid was performed once more on admission to the department of surgery just before the thyroidectomy or during visit in an outpatient clinic after the results of the biopsy were obtained or during the qualification for thyroidectomy. The ultrasound examinations were carried out using a Samsung RS80 EVO device (Samsung Medison, Seoul, Korea) with a 3–12 MHz linear array probe (L3-12A). CAD in our study was based on K-TIRADS classification and using S-Detect 2 software (Samsung Medison Co. Ltd., Seoul, South Korea). The following ultrasound features were assessed automatically: composition (partially cystic, solid, or cystic), echogenity (hyper/isoechoic or hypoechoic), orientation (parallel or non-parallel), margin (ill-defined, well-defined smooth, or microlobulated/spiculated), spongiform (appearance or nonappearance), shape (ovoid to round or irregular), and calcifications (microcalcification, macrocalcification, or no calcification), which were automatically assessed by the US device. Elasticity and vascularity were not assessed by CAD and have not been taken into consideration for risk stratification, because they had to be introduced manually, while for our study we intended to check the performance of CAD without being distracted by any features that were operator-dependent. Each nodule was eventually classified by S-Detect into two categories: possibly benign and possibly malignant.

The ultrasound examinations were conducted at the Department of Endocrinology, Metabolism, and Internal Medicine of Poznan University of Medical Sciences in Poznan, Poland, and at the Department of Oncological Endocrinology and Nuclear Medicine at Maria Sklodowska-Curie National Research Institute of Oncology in Warsaw, Poland. During the ultrasound examination, the transverse and longitudinal planes for both the gland and the nodules were obtained while the patient was in the supine position. The anteroposterior, transverse, and longitudinal diameters of the nodules were measured on frozen images during examination and then archived.

The examinations were performed by four physicians with at least 10 years of experience in thyroid ultrasound examination and working at the departments specialized in diagnostics and treatment of thyroid cancer. The nodules were classified with an EU-TIRADS score independently by two physicians on the basis of recorded examinations. In seven cases, there was disagreement with the score by one point. The consensus on the final grade was made together after discussion. Physicians evaluating the EU-TIRADS score were blinded to the biopsy results and/or histopathological examination. All nodules were scored according to the European Thyroid Association Guidelines for Ultrasound Malignancy Risk Stratification of Thyroid Nodules in Adults [7]. EU-TIRADS was used in a pattern-based model, where we assessed only the above-mentioned ultrasound features.

2.2.2. Statistical Analysis

The calculations were performed with Statistica 12 (TIBCO Software Inc., Palo Alto, CA 94304, USA). The p-value < 0.05 was considered significant. Sensitivities, specificities, positive and negative predictive values, and diagnostic accuracies were calculated to assess S-Detect and the EU-TIRADS scale. Comparisons of the diagnostic values of the tests were done using McNemar's test. EU-TIRADS classes 4 and 5 were considered as positive, whereas classes 1 to 3 were considered as negative (MODELS 1–3); in MODELS 4 and 5, only EU-TIRADS class 5 was considered as positive. Moreover, "possible malignant" by S-Detect corresponded to a positive result, whereas "possibly benign" corresponded to a negative result. The histopathological and cytological examinations served as a reference for a true or a false result.

2.2.3. Ethical Approval

The study was approved by the institutional bioethical review board of each participating institution where the patients were examined, namely Poznan University of Medical Sciences and Maria Sklodowska-Curie National Research Institute of Oncology, both in Poland. All procedures were in accordance with the ethical standards of the institutional and/or national research committee and with the 1964 Helsinki Declaration and its later amendments or comparable ethical standards. Informed consent was obtained from all patients participating in the study to publish this report.

3. Results

Eighty-eight patients (70 women, 18 men) aged 49.4 ± 15.5 (17–80) years with 133 thyroid lesions were included in the study; of these, fifty-eight patients were diagnosed with 66 malignant lesions (including 57 papillary thyroid cancers (PTCs), four follicular variants of PTC, two medullary thyroid cancers (MTCs), one follicular thyroid cancer (FTC), two nodules in one patient described as poorly differentiated thyroid cancer). Benign lesions were colloid or hyperplastic nodules. The results of the diagnostic value of CAD-based S-Detect and physician-based EU-TIRADS (lesions with the score 4 or 5 were regarded as suspected for malignancy) are presented in Table 1. There was a statistically significant difference in the performance of CAD-based S-Detect and physician-based EU-TIRADS ($p = 0.009$).

Table 1. Results for the assessment of thyroid lesions using S-Detect only, the European Thyroid Imaging Reporting and Data System (EU-TIRADS) scale (4 and 5 points), and the mixed MODELs 1 to 5.

Groups	Sensitivity		Specificity		PPV		NPV		Accuracy	
	Value	95% CI	Value	95% CI	Value	95% CI	Value	95% CI	Value	95% CI
S-Detect	89.4	79.4–95.6	80.6	69.1–89.2	81.9	73.5–88.2	88.5	79.1–94.0	85.0	77.7–90.6
EU-TIRADS (4 and 5 points)	90.9	81.3–96.6	61.2	48.5–72.9	69.8	62.9–75.9	87.2	75.7–93.8	75.9	67.8–82.9
EU-TIRADS (5 points)	80.0	68.7–88.6	79.4	67.9–88.3	80.0	71.2–86.6	79.4	70.4–86.2	79.7	72.0–86.1
MODEL 1	84.9	73–92.5	88.1	77.8–94.7	87.5	78.4–93.1	85.5	76.8–91.3	86.5	79.5–91.8
MODEL 2	95.5	87.3–99.1	53.7	41.1–66.0	67.0	61.0–72.6	92.3	79.5–97.4	74.4	66.2–81.6
MODEL 3	93.9	85.2–98.3	73.1	60.9–83.2	77.5	69.8–83.7	92.5	82.4–97.0	83.5	76.0–89.3
MODEL 4	78.9	67.0–87.9	89.6	79.7–95.7	88.1	78.5–93.8	81.1	72.8–87.3	84.2	76.9–90.0
MODEL 5	93.9	85.2–98.3	80.6	69.1–89.2	82.7	74.5–88.6	93.1	83.8–97.2	87.2	80.3–92.4

CI, confidence interval; PPV, positive predictive value; NPV, negative predictive value; EU-TIRADS, European Thyroid Imaging Reporting and Data System.

Next, we structured five models using both CAD-based S-Detect and physician-based EU-TIRADS (Table 2).

Table 2. Description of the mixed models. The S-Detect classification was based on computer-aided diagnosis (CAD). The nodules were classified with an European Thyroid Imaging Reporting and Data System (EU-TIRADS) score independently by two physicians on the basis of recorded examinations.

	EU-TIRADS Scale		S-Detect Classification
MODEL 1	4 or 5 points	AND	"possibly malignant"
MODEL 2	4 or 5 points	OR	"possibly malignant"
MODEL 3	5 points	-	-
	3 or 4 points	AND	"possibly malignant"
MODEL 4	5 points	AND	"possibly malignant"
MODEL 5	5 points	OR	"possibly malignant"

MODEL 1 assumes that:
- a suspected lesion obtains 4 or 5 points on the EU-TIRADS scale

and
- is classified by S-Detect as "possibly malignant".

A significant difference between the diagnostic efficacy of MODEL 1 and EU-TIRADS ($p < 0.0001$) as well as MODEL 1 and S-Detect ($p = 0.013$) was detected. The diagnostic effectiveness of MODEL 1 is presented in Table 1 (row 4).

MODEL 2 was based on the assumption that:
- a suspected lesion obtains 4 or 5 points on the EU-TIRADS scale

or
- is classified as "possibly malignant" by S-Detect (Table 1, row 5).

There was no statistically significant difference between MODEL 2 and the EU-TIRADS scale alone ($p = 0.13$), whereas MODEL 2 performed significantly worse than S-Detect itself ($p < 0.001$).

MODEL 3 was based on the assumption that:
- a suspected lesion obtains 5 points on the EU-TIRADS scale

or
- obtains 3 or 4 points on the EU-TIRADS scale **and** simultaneously is classified as "possibly malignant" by S-Detect (Table 1, row 6).

MODEL 4 assumes that:
- a suspected lesion obtains 5 points on the EU-TIRADS scale

and
- is classified by S-Detect as "possibly malignant" (Table 1, row 7).

There was no significant difference ($p > 0.05$) between the accuracy of MODEL 4 and the similar MODEL 1, however the sensitivity was slightly lower with better specificity.

MODEL 5 was based on the assumption that:
- a suspected lesion obtains 5 points on the EU-TIRADS scale

or
- is classified as "possibly malignant" by S-Detect (Table 1, row 8).

There was no significant difference between the results of MODEL 5 and the similarly constructed MODEL 2 ($p > 0.05$).

The overall diagnostic performance of MODEL 3 is also not statistically significantly different from the EU-TIRADS scale alone ($p = 0.26$) but is slightly worse ($p < 0.027$) than S-Detect alone (Table 1, row 5). The obtained results suggest the superiority of MODEL 1 over the other two models as well as over the EU-TIRADS scale or S-Detect used separately. Table 2 summarizes the details of the approach used for each MODEL. Figure 2 presents an example of two lesions that were diagnosed in one patient and whose character was correctly predicted by S-Detect. The first lesion was given 4 points on the EU-TIRADS scale and was diagnosed as "possibly malignant" by S-Detect, whereas the final histopathological examination revealed the malignant character of the lesion (medullary thyroid cancer). The second lesion, although it may be attributed as suspected due to its taller-than-wide shape, was diagnosed as "possibly benign" by S-Detect, whereas it eventually turned out to be a benign hyperplastic nodule.

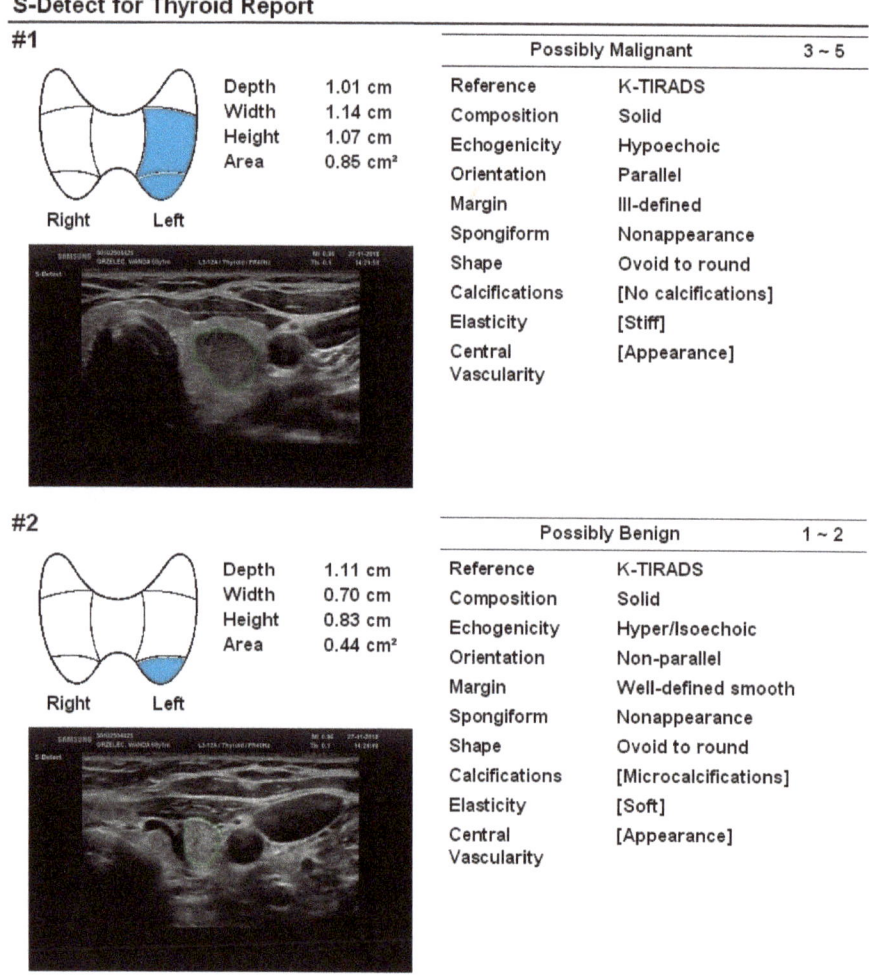

Figure 2. Two lesions diagnosed in one patient. The first lesion obtains 4 points on the EU-TIRADS scale, was diagnosed as "possibly malignant" by S-Detect, and the final histopathological examination revealed the malignant character of the lesion (medullary thyroid cancer). The second lesion, although it may be attributed as suspected due to its taller-than-wide shape was diagnosed as "possibly benign" by S-Detect, whereas it eventually turned out to be a benign hyperplastic nodule. Only features assessed automatically by the device, as the operator-independent ones were taken into consideration in the S-Detect classification. The two last features—elasticity and central vascularity—were not included in the S-Detect prediction. K-TIRADS, Korean Thyroid Imaging Reporting and Data System.

4. Discussion

Since 2009, when the first two classifications of TIRADS lexicons (Horvath and Park) were elaborated, there has been an ongoing struggle to improve the accuracy of the evaluation of TNs that would result in the adequate referral for FNAB [19]. This problem is very complicated in nature due to the diverse ultrasound features of malignant TNs and also to their different oncological aggressiveness. The performance of different classification systems also depends on the population groups being examined (i.e., oncological patients vs. primary center patients). We presume that our study satisfies the high demand for evaluating the new and promising systems and the combination of these systems for TN differentiation. To the best of our knowledge, this study constitutes the unique dual-center analysis comparing the diagnostic performance of S-Detect software and the EU-TIRADS classification in predicting the character of TNs. EU-TIRADS was established to improve inter-observer reproducibility and to facilitate communication between medical physicians [7,20]. Recent studies have demonstrated that, when using the EU-TIRADS classification, the sensitivity is satisfactory, but specificity might still be insufficient. Dobruch-Sobczak et al. have reported 98.7% sensitivity, 39.8% specificity, 38.0% PPV, and 98.8% NPV in nodules assessed as EU-TIRADS ≥4 [12]. Comparable results were obtained by Schenke et al. for small thyroid nodules (<10 mm) and presented as follows: 97.4%, 49.3%, 67.9%, and 94.4%, respectively [21]. However, Skowronska et al. indicated the following values of the mentioned parameters: 75.0%, 94.1%, 75.0%, and 94.1%, respectively, taking into account a similar threshold for the EU-TIRADS score as indicating suspected lesions [22]. In our current prospective study, the obtained value for sensitivity was high and equal to 90.9%. The specificity was moderately satisfactory and reached 61.2%. The results obtained for PPV and NPV were acceptable and similar to those in previous studies indicating that PPV of the scale is lower than NPV (69.8% and 87.2%, respectively). In this context, EU-TIRADS should be used rather to exclude malignancy (or indicate the TNs of very low probability of thyroid cancer), and those nodules might be only followed up without biopsy. On the other hand, lesions obtaining a high score on this scale should be qualified for biopsy, which is still considered as the gold standard of TN diagnostics and the most important basis of clinical decision-making in patients with TNs.

Differentiation between benign and malignant TNs is challenging, even for experienced specialists. Accordingly, some recent studies have focused on S-Detect system efficacy in comparison to evaluations performed by experienced medical physicians or other types of evaluations using CAD [14,15]. A recent meta-analysis performed by Zhao et al. including 723 lesions from five studies revealed that the sensitivity of the CAD was comparable to the assessment provided by experienced radiologists (0.87 vs. 0.88) but presented lower specificity (0.79 vs. 0.92). However, there is a need for larger sample-size prospective studies to verify the clinical usefulness of CAD in a clinical setting, together with further technical improvements of the software [15].

S-Detect for thyroid is a newly developed advanced technological tool aimed at improving the non-invasive classification of TNs. This CAD is alternatively based on the Korean Thyroid Imaging Reporting and Data System (K-TIRADS), the Russian TIRADS (RUSS) and the American Thyroid Association (ATA) guidelines. Recent meta-analyses have been focused on considerable discrepancies across ultrasound risk stratification systems and their diagnostic performance. The overall diagnostic performance of the four US-based risk stratification systems was comparable [23]. The present meta-analysis found a higher performance of American Collage of Radiology TIRADS (ACR-TIRADS) in selecting thyroid nodules for FNAB. However, the comparison across the most common US reporting systems was limited by the data available. Further studies are needed to confirm this finding [13].

Gitto et al. in their retrospective study, involving 62 patients, compared the diagnostic performance of CAD and that obtained by radiologists. The sensitivity was relatively low for CAD and equal to 21.4%, and was significantly lower than the sensitivity obtained by radiologists (78.6%). In contrast, our study demonstrated high sensitivity of S-Detect (89.4%), comparable to the assessment made by experienced sonographers using the EU-TIRADS scale (90.9%). With respect to specificity, no significant difference between CAD and radiologists was observed [24]. In our study, the specificity of S-Detect

(80.6%) was also quite high and better than that of the experienced sonographers (61.2%). A high NPV of S-Detect (78.0%) together with a low PPV (25.0%) were indicated by Gitto et al. [24]. We obtained a slightly higher value for NPV; however, PPV was much more satisfactory according to our results (81.9%). In our group, assessing the malignancy risk using the EU-TIRADS scale had a lower PPV and a similar NPV in comparison to S-Detect. In terms of diagnostic accuracy, Gitto et al. observed quite similar values for S-Detect and radiologists (67.7% and 69.4%, respectively). According to our results, both values were higher (85% for S-Detect and 75.9 for endocrinologists using the EU-TIRADS scale). However, the accuracy was even better when S-Detect was combined with the EU-TIRADS assessment (86.5%). In contrast, Kim et al. in their retrospective analysis encompassing 218 nodules in 106 patients showed similar sensitivity (81.4% vs. 84.9%), but lower specificity (68.2% vs. 96.2%) of S-Detect 2, if compared to radiologists [25]. In agreement with our study, PPV of S-Detect was lower than NPV [25]. Other clinical studies showed comparable results of sensitivity (88.6%–92.0%) and specificity (74.6–87.9%) if compared to our results [26–29]. In the literature, PPV ranges from 57.5% to 89.2% [26–29], which is in agreement with our results (81.9%). We indicated slightly lower, but still satisfactory NPV (88.5%) than previous authors (90.4–98.4%) [26–29]. The discordant results, that is, low specificity (41.2%) and high sensitivity (90.5%) in the detection of malignant TNs, was reported by Xia et al. in their prospective study performed in a specialized thyroid center including 180 lesions [30]. In another study by Yoo et al. including 50 patients with 117 nodules, the authors indicated that the diagnostic performance of CAD was similar to that of radiologists [9]. It is worth noting that, similarly to our study, the authors indicated a quite high PPV (83.3%). In addition, CAD-assisted radiologists performed better in terms of sensitivity than radiologists alone [9]. This is in agreement with our study, which indicated that the combined model of taking into consideration both S-Detect and the EU-TIRADS scale assessment is better than either approach alone.

The only study performed in a similar population to ours (but including a lower number of lesions) was the one by Barczyński et al. They found that the overall accuracy of S-Detect was 82% if compared to 76% for the assessment by a surgeon with basic skills. However, the authors simultaneously indicated that CAD was inferior to an expert surgeon, due to six false-positive results [16]. A similar conclusion can be derived from the study by Chung et al. [27], where CAD performed better than a less experienced radiologist, while at least as good as an experienced physician. The summary of previous studies that evaluated the diagnostic performance of S-Detect is presented in Table 3. The results of our prospective study indicated that the evaluation of TNs based on EU-TIRADS is associated with comparable sensitivity (90.9% vs. 89.4%), but much lower specificity (61.2% vs. 80.6%) than analysis performed by S-Detect. In terms of PPV and NPV, the former is significantly better for S-Detect (81.9% vs. 69.8%), while NPV is comparable for EU-TIRADS and S-Detect used separately (87.2% vs. 88.5%). However, the combination of S-Detect and EU-TIRADS allows to maintain high sensitivity (84.9%), while, importantly, it improves specificity (up to 88.1%) as obtained for MODEL 1 in comparison to EU-TIRADS itself (61.2%). Thus, we can conclude that the evaluation of TNs using the EU-TIRADS scale by an experienced sonographer and the simultaneous evaluation by S-Detect may be complementary methods and should optimally be used together.

Table 3. Comparison of diagnostic performance of the computer-aided diagnosis (CAD) system and experienced staff.

	Number of Patients	Number of Nodules	Sensitivity (%)		Specificity (%)		PPV (%)		NPV (%)		Accuracy (%)	
			CAD	Staff	CAD	Staff	CAD	Staff	CAD	Staff	CAD	Staff
**Current study *, ** **	**88**	**133**	**89.4**	**90.9**	**80.6**	**61.2**	**81.9**	**69.8**	**88.5**	**87.2**	**85.0**	**75.9**
Gitto S et al.	62	62	21.4	78.6	81.3	66.7	25.0	40.7	78	91.4	67.7	69.4
Kim HL et al. *	106	218	81.4	84.9	68.2	96.2	62.5	93.6	84.9	90.7	73.4	91.7
Jeong EY et al.	85	100	88.6	84.1	83.9	96.4	81.3	94.9	90.4	88.5	86.0	91.0
Chung SR et al. **	197	197	92.0	84.0	87.9	97.9	57.5	87.5	98.4	97.2	88.5	95.8
Park VY et al.	265	286	90.4–91.0	94.2	58.5–80.0	76.9	72.3–84.5	83.1	83.5–88.1	91.7	75.9–86.0	86.4
Choi YJ et al.	89	102	90.7	88.4	74.6	94.9	72.2	92.7	91.7	91.8	81.4	92.2
Xia S et al.	171	180	90.5	81.1	41.2	88.5	63.2	6.7	79.5	95.9	67.2	60.9

* CAD, only S-Detect 2 was taken into account. ** Staff with ≥7 years of experience. CAD, computer-aided diagnosis; PPV, positive predictive value; NPV, negative predictive value.

The lack of the histopathological verification of 35 nodules should be mentioned here as a potential limitation of the study. Of these, 17 were not subjected to surgical procedure due to a benign cytological character, an unsuspicious ultrasound picture, and a lack of local symptoms (large goiter, compressive symptoms, dysphagia, dysphonia).

5. Conclusions

S-Detect software characterizes with high sensitivity and good specificity, and may thus be useful in screening for suspected lesions by less experienced sonographers. The EU-TIRADS classification allows to identify suspected lesions with high sensitivity but rather low specificity. The best diagnostic performance in malignant thyroid nodule (TN) risk stratification was obtained for the combined model of S-Detect ("possibly malignant" nodule) and simultaneously obtaining 4 or 5 points (MODEL 1) or exactly 5 points (MODEL 5) on the EU-TIRADS scale.

Author Contributions: Conceptualization, E.S.-P., K.W. and M.R.; methodology, K.D.-S., B.M., R.Z.S., A.K., A.Z. and Z.A.; validation, E.S.-P., K.W. and K.D.S.; resources, M.L.-R. and T.B.; writing—original draft preparation, P.A. and A.O.; writing—review and editing, E.S.-P., K.W. and K.D.-S.; visualization, R.Z.S. and R.K.M.; supervision, M.D., A.L. and M.R. All authors have read and agreed to the published version of the manuscript.

Funding: This research received no external funding.

Conflicts of Interest: The authors declare no conflict of interest.

References

1. Wolinski, K.; Stangierski, A.; Ruchala, M. Comparison of diagnostic yield of core-needle and fine-needle aspiration biopsies of thyroid lesions: Systematic review and meta-analysis. *Eur. Radiol.* **2017**, *27*, 431–436. [CrossRef] [PubMed]
2. Tumino, D.; Grani, G.; Di Stefano, M.; Di Mauro, M.; Scutari, M.; Rago, T.; Fugazzola, L.; Castagna, M.G.; Maino, F. Nodular Thyroid Disease in the Era of Precision Medicine. *Front. Endocrinol. (Lausanne)* **2019**, *10*, 907. [CrossRef] [PubMed]
3. Ruchala, M.; Szczepanek, E. Thyroid ultrasound—A piece of cake? *Endokrynol. Pol.* **2010**, *61*, 330–344. [PubMed]
4. Szczepanek-Parulska, E.; Wolinski, K.; Stangierski, A.; Gurgul, E.; Biczysko, M.; Majewski, P.; Rewaj-Losyk, M.; Ruchala, M. Comparison of diagnostic value of conventional ultrasonography and shear wave elastography in the prediction of thyroid lesions malignancy. *PLoS ONE* **2013**, *8*, e81532. [CrossRef]
5. Dobruch-Sobczak, K.; Migda, B.; Krauze, A.; Mlosek, K.; Slapa, R.Z.; Wareluk, P.; Bakula-Zalewska, E.; Adamczewski, Z.; Lewinski, A.; Jakubowski, W.; et al. Prospective analysis of inter-observer and intra-observer variability in multi ultrasound descriptor assessment of thyroid nodules. *J. Ultrason.* **2019**, *19*, 198–206. [CrossRef]
6. Wolinski, K.; Szkudlarek, M.; Szczepanek-Parulska, E.; Ruchala, M. Usefulness of different ultrasound features of malignancy in predicting the type of thyroid lesions: A meta-analysis of prospective studies. *Pol. Arch. Med. Wewn.* **2014**, *124*, 97–104. [CrossRef]
7. Russ, G.; Bonnema, S.J.; Erdogan, M.F.; Durante, C.; Ngu, R.; Leenhardt, L. European Thyroid Association Guidelines for Ultrasound Malignancy Risk Stratification of Thyroid Nodules in Adults: The EU-TIRADS. *Eur. Thyroid. J.* **2017**, *6*, 225–237. [CrossRef]
8. Jin, Z.; Zhu, Y.; Zhang, S.; Xie, F.; Zhang, M.; Zhang, Y.; Tian, X.; Zhang, J.; Luo, Y.; Cao, J. Ultrasound Computer-Aided Diagnosis (CAD) Based on the Thyroid Imaging Reporting and Data System (TI-RADS) to Distinguish Benign from Malignant Thyroid Nodules and the Diagnostic Performance of Radiologists with Different Diagnostic Experience. *Med. Sci. Monit.* **2020**, *26*, e918452. [CrossRef]
9. Yoo, Y.J.; Ha, E.J.; Cho, Y.J.; Kim, H.L.; Han, M.; Kang, S.Y. Computer-Aided Diagnosis of Thyroid Nodules via Ultrasonography: Initial Clinical Experience. *Korean J. Radiol.* **2018**, *19*, 665–672. [CrossRef]
10. Luo, J.; Huang, F.; Zhou, P.; Chen, J.; Sun, Y.; Xu, F.; Wu, L.; Huang, P. Is ultrasound combined with computed tomography useful for distinguishing between primary thyroid lymphoma and Hashimoto's thyroiditis? *Endokrynol. Pol.* **2019**, *70*, 463–468. [CrossRef]

11. Dobruch-Sobczak, K.S.; Krauze, A.; Migda, B.; Mlosek, K.; Slapa, R.Z.; Bakula-Zalewska, E.; Adamczewski, Z.; Lewinski, A.; Jakubowski, W.; Dedecjus, M. Integration of Sonoelastography Into the TIRADS Lexicon Could Influence the Classification. *Front. Endocrinol. (Lausanne)* **2019**, *10*, 127. [CrossRef]
12. Dobruch-Sobczak, K.; Adamczewski, Z.; Szczepanek-Parulska, E.; Migda, B.; Wolinski, K.; Krauze, A.; Prostko, P.; Ruchala, M.; Lewinski, A.; Jakubowski, W.; et al. Histopathological Verification of the Diagnostic Performance of the EU-TIRADS Classification of Thyroid Nodules-Results of a Multicenter Study Performed in a Previously Iodine-Deficient Region. *J. Clin. Med.* **2019**, *8*, 1781. [CrossRef] [PubMed]
13. Castellana, M.; Grani, G.; Radzina, M.; Guerra, V.; Giovanella, L.; Deandrea, M.; Ngu, R.; Durante, C.; Trimboli, P. Performance of EU-TIRADS in malignancy risk stratification of thyroid nodules. A meta-analysis. *Eur. J. Endocrinol.* **2020**. [CrossRef] [PubMed]
14. Chambara, N.; Ying, M. The Diagnostic Efficiency of Ultrasound Computer-Aided Diagnosis in Differentiating Thyroid Nodules: A Systematic Review and Narrative Synthesis. *Cancers (Basel)* **2019**, *11*, 1759. [CrossRef]
15. Zhao, W.J.; Fu, L.R.; Huang, Z.M.; Zhu, J.Q.; Ma, B.Y. Effectiveness evaluation of computer-aided diagnosis system for the diagnosis of thyroid nodules on ultrasound: A systematic review and meta-analysis. *Medicine (Baltimore)* **2019**, *98*, e16349. [CrossRef]
16. Barczynski, M.; Stopa-Barczynska, M.; Wojtczak, B.; Czarniecka, A.; Konturek, A. Clinical validation of S-Detect(TM) mode in semi-automated ultrasound classification of thyroid lesions in surgical office. *Gland Surg.* **2020**, *9*, S77–S85. [CrossRef]
17. Migda, B.; Migda, M.; Migda, M.S.; Slapa, R.Z. Use of the Kwak Thyroid Image Reporting and Data System (K-TIRADS) in differential diagnosis of thyroid nodules: Systematic review and meta-analysis. *Eur. Radiol.* **2018**, *28*, 2380–2388. [CrossRef]
18. Fresilli, D.; Grani, G.; De Pascali, M.L.; Alagna, G.; Tassone, E.; Ramundo, V.; Ascoli, V.; Bosco, D.; Biffoni, M.; Bononi, M.; et al. Computer-aided diagnostic system for thyroid nodule sonographic evaluation outperforms the specificity of less experienced examiners. *J. Ultrasound.* **2020**, *23*, 169–174. [CrossRef]
19. Migda, B.; Migda, M.; Migda, A.M.; Bierca, J.; Slowniska-Srzednicka, J.; Jakubowski, W.; Slapa, R.Z. Evaluation of Four Variants of the Thyroid Imaging Reporting and Data System (TIRADS) Classification in Patients with Multinodular Goitre—Initial study. *Endokrynol. Pol.* **2018**, *69*, 156–162. [CrossRef]
20. Grani, G.; Lamartina, L.; Cantisani, V.; Maranghi, M.; Lucia, P.; Durante, C. Interobserver agreement of various thyroid imaging reporting and data systems. *Endocr. Connect.* **2018**, *7*, 1–7. [CrossRef]
21. Schenke, S.; Klett, R.; Seifert, P.; Kreissl, M.C.; Gorges, R.; Zimny, M. Diagnostic Performance of Different Thyroid Imaging Reporting and Data Systems (Kwak-TIRADS, EU-TIRADS and ACR TI-RADS) for Risk Stratification of Small Thyroid Nodules (≤10 mm). *J. Clin. Med.* **2020**, *9*, 236. [CrossRef]
22. Skowronska, A.; Milczarek-Banach, J.; Wiechno, W.; Chudzinski, W.; Zach, M.; Mazurkiewicz, M.; Miskiewicz, P.; Bednarczuk, T. Accuracy of the European Thyroid Imaging Reporting and Data System (EU-TIRADS) in the valuation of thyroid nodule malignancy in reference to the post-surgery histological results. *Pol. J. Radiol.* **2018**, *83*, e579–e586. [CrossRef] [PubMed]
23. Kim, P.H.; Suh, C.H.; Baek, J.H.; Chung, S.R.; Choi, Y.J.; Lee, J.H. Diagnostic Performance of Four Ultrasound Risk Stratification Systems: A Systematic Review and Meta-Analysis. *Thyroid* **2020**. [CrossRef] [PubMed]
24. Gitto, S.; Grassi, G.; De Angelis, C.; Monaco, C.G.; Sdao, S.; Sardanelli, F.; Sconfienza, L.M.; Mauri, G. A computer-aided diagnosis system for the assessment and characterization of low-to-high suspicion thyroid nodules on ultrasound. *Radiol. Med.* **2019**, *124*, 118–125. [CrossRef]
25. Kim, H.L.; Ha, E.J.; Han, M. Real-World Performance of Computer-Aided Diagnosis System for Thyroid Nodules Using Ultrasonography. *Ultrasound. Med. Biol.* **2019**, *45*, 2672–2678. [CrossRef]
26. Jeong, E.Y.; Kim, H.L.; Ha, E.J.; Park, S.Y.; Cho, Y.J.; Han, M. Computer-aided diagnosis system for thyroid nodules on ultrasonography: Diagnostic performance and reproducibility based on the experience level of operators. *Eur. Radiol.* **2019**, *29*, 1978–1985. [CrossRef]
27. Chung, S.R.; Baek, J.H.; Lee, M.K.; Ahn, Y.; Choi, Y.J.; Sung, T.Y.; Song, D.E.; Kim, T.Y.; Lee, J.H. Computer-Aided Diagnosis System for the Evaluation of Thyroid Nodules on Ultrasonography: Prospective Non-Inferiority Study according to the Experience Level of Radiologists. *Korean J. Radiol.* **2020**, *21*, 369–376. [CrossRef]
28. Park, V.Y.; Han, K.; Seong, Y.K.; Park, M.H.; Kim, E.K.; Moon, H.J.; Yoon, J.H.; Kwak, J.Y. Diagnosis of Thyroid Nodules: Performance of a Deep Learning Convolutional Neural Network Model vs. Radiologists. *Sci. Rep.* **2019**, *9*, 17843. [CrossRef]

29. Choi, Y.J.; Baek, J.H.; Park, H.S.; Shim, W.H.; Kim, T.Y.; Shong, Y.K.; Lee, J.H. A Computer-Aided Diagnosis System Using Artificial Intelligence for the Diagnosis and Characterization of Thyroid Nodules on Ultrasound: Initial Clinical Assessment. *Thyroid* **2017**, *27*, 546–552. [CrossRef]
30. Xia, S.; Yao, J.; Zhou, W.; Dong, Y.; Xu, S.; Zhou, J.; Zhan, W. A computer-aided diagnosing system in the evaluation of thyroid nodules-experience in a specialized thyroid center. *World J. Surg. Oncol.* **2019**, *17*, 210. [CrossRef]

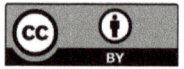

© 2020 by the authors. Licensee MDPI, Basel, Switzerland. This article is an open access article distributed under the terms and conditions of the Creative Commons Attribution (CC BY) license (http://creativecommons.org/licenses/by/4.0/).

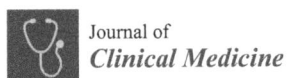

Article

Detection of BRAFV600E in Liquid Biopsy from Patients with Papillary Thyroid Cancer Is Associated with Tumor Aggressiveness and Response to Therapy

Kirk Jensen [1], Shilpa Thakur [2], Aneeta Patel [1], Maria Cecilia Mendonca-Torres [1], John Costello [1], Cristiane Jeyce Gomes-Lima [2,3], Mary Walter [2], Leonard Wartofsky [3], Kenneth Dale Burman [3], Athanasios Bikas [3], Dorina Ylli [1,4], Vasyl V. Vasko [1] and Joanna Klubo-Gwiezdzinska [2,*]

1. Department of Pediatrics, Endocrine Division, Uniformed Services University of the Health Sciences, Bethesda, MD 20814, USA; kirk.jensen@usuhs.edu (K.J.); aneeta.patel@usuhs.edu (A.P.); maria.mendonca-torres@usuhs.edu (M.C.M.-T.); john.costello.ctr@usuhs.edu (J.C.); dorina.ylli@umed.edu.al (D.Y.); vasyl.vasko.ctr@usuhs.edu (V.V.V.)
2. National Institute of Diabetes and Digestive and Kidney Diseases, National Institutes of Health, Bethesda, MD 20814, USA; shilpa.thakur@nih.gov (S.T.); cjglima@gmail.com (C.J.G.-L.); waltermf@niddk.nih.gov (M.W.)
3. MedStar Health Research Institute, MedStar Washington Hospital Center, Washington, DC 20010, USA; leonard.wartofsky@medstar.net (L.W.); Kenneth.D.Burman@medstar.net (K.D.B.); athanasiosbikas@gmail.com (A.B.)
4. Endocrinology Division, University of Medicine, 1005 Tirana, Albania
* Correspondence: joanna.klubogwiezdzinska@nih.gov; Tel.: +301-496-5052

Received: 19 June 2020; Accepted: 30 July 2020; Published: 2 August 2020

Abstract: The detection of rare mutational targets in plasma (liquid biopsy) has emerged as a promising tool for the assessment of patients with cancer. We determined the presence of cell-free DNA containing the *BRAFV600E* mutations (cf*BRAFV600E*) in plasma samples from 57 patients with papillary thyroid cancer (PTC) with somatic *BRAFV600E* mutation-positive primary tumors using microfluidic digital PCR, and co-amplification at lower denaturation temperature (COLD) PCR. Mutant cf*BRAFV600E* alleles were detected in 24/57 (42.1%) of the examined patients. The presence of cf*BRAFV600E* was significantly associated with tumor size ($p = 0.03$), multifocal patterns of growth ($p = 0.03$), the presence of extrathyroidal gross extension ($p = 0.02$) and the presence of pulmonary micrometastases ($p = 0.04$). In patients with low-, intermediate- and high-risk PTCs, cf*BRAFV600E* was detected in 4/19 (21.0%), 8/22 (36.3%) and 12/16 (75.0%) of cases, respectively. Patients with detectable cf*BRAFV600E* were characterized by a 4.68 times higher likelihood of non-excellent response to therapy, as compared to patients without detectable cf*BRAF*V600E (OR (odds ratios), 4.68; 95% CI (confidence intervals)) 1.26–17.32; $p = 0.02$). In summary, the combination of digital polymerase chain reaction (dPCR) with COLD-PCR enables the detection of *BRAFV600E* in the liquid biopsy from patients with PTCs and could prove useful for the identification of patients with PTC at an increased risk for a structurally or biochemically incomplete or indeterminate response to treatment.

Keywords: COLD-PCR; digital PCR; *BRAFV600E*; papillary thyroid cancer; liquid biopsy

1. Introduction

Advances in the understanding of genetic and biologic characteristics of thyroid cancer, coupled with the development of new molecular targeted therapeutics, have led to improved diagnosis and treatment [1]. Progress in the characterization of the genomic landscape of thyroid cancers was principally fostered through next-generation sequencing (NGS) methods, allowing the detection of multiple variants simultaneously, including base substitutions, insertion/deletions, gene amplifications and gene rearrangements [2]. The analysis of genomic variants revealed a high frequency of activating somatic alterations of genes encoding effectors in the mitogen-activated protein kinase (MAPK) signaling pathway, including the point mutations of *BRAF* and the *RAS* genes, as well as fusions involving the RET and NTRK1 tyrosine kinases. *BRAF* mutations have been the most frequently detected genomic alterations in papillary thyroid cancer (PTC), being primarily mutations encoding V600E substitution [2–4].

On average, the frequency of the *BRAFV600E* mutation is 45% in PTC patients, but its prevalence can vary from 25–82% depending on the population examined [5,6]. The presence of *BRAFV600E* mutation in PTC patients has been associated with increased tumor progression, aggressive clinicopathological features and poorer prognosis, particularly when coupled with a telomerase reverse transcriptase (TERT) promoter mutation. Specifically, adverse clinical-pathological features associated with the *BRAFV600E* mutation include the presence of lymph node metastases, extrathyroidal invasion, distant metastases and advanced cancer stages [3,7]. Moreover, the occurrence of the *BRAFV600E* mutation has been correlated with tumor recurrence and reduced or absent radioiodine (RAI) avidity, leading to the failure of RAI therapy [8]. A linear relationship has also been observed between patient age and mortality risk in PTC patients with *BRAFV600E* mutation [3,9,10].

The detection of the *BRAFV600E* mutation in thyroid cancer patients has been conventionally determined by fine-needle aspiration (FNA) or tissue biopsy, followed by molecular testing and/or immunohistochemistry [11,12]. Growing evidence demonstrates that blood-based liquid biopsies provide a minimally invasive alternative for identifying the cellular and molecular signatures that can be used as biomarkers to detect early-stage cancer and predict disease progression [13,14]. In this context, the examination of circulating cell-free *BRAFV600E* (cf*BRAFV600E*) in blood could represent an attractive approach for diagnosis and monitoring the response to treatment in patients with PTC.

Since the amounts of cfDNA and cfRNA in blood are low, highly sensitive techniques are required for genomic analysis in liquid biopsy. Polymerase chain reaction (PCR) coupled with direct sequencing is a standard method for the detection of mutations, but this method is not sufficiently sensitive for the detection of low levels of DNA variants in a mixture of wild type and mutant sequences. Currently, droplet digital PCR (dPCR) is considered the technique of choice for the detection of rare mutations in liquid biopsy samples [15–18]. Recent studies demonstrated that dPCR can be successfully employed for monitoring response to therapy by quantifying *BRAF* and *RAS* mutants in samples from patients with cancers [19–21]. Another approach applies the techniques that allow the enrichment of low abundance variants in DNA samples. Co-amplification at lower denaturation temperature-based PCR (COLD-PCR) is a modified PCR method that allows the preferential amplification of rare mutant alleles within a target amplicon [22–24]. The unique attribute of COLD-PCR is that the selective enrichment of low-abundance mutations within a target amplicon is achieved by exploiting a small difference in the amplicon melting temperature [25,26]. Recent studies demonstrated that COLD-PCR was 10–100 times more sensitive than standard PCR in the detection of mutant variants. Currently, various versions of COLD-PCR (full-, ice-, fast-, TT-COLD-PCR) have been developed and utilized successfully for the detection of mutated genes, including *KRAS*, *HRAS*, *NRAS*, *EGFR*, *TP53* and *BRAF* [23,24,27].

Until now, no data have demonstrated the suitability of the COLD-PCR method in the detection of a *BRAFV600E* mutation in liquid biopsy samples from thyroid cancer patients. In the current study, we investigated the utility of COLD-PCR in combination with digital PCR for the detection of *BRAFV600E* in liquid biopsy samples from the patients with PTC. The data derived were utilized to analyze the potential utility of this approach to improve the risk stratification and response to treatment in patients with thyroid cancer.

2. Materials and Methods

2.1. Subjects

This study was approved by the Uniformed Service University of the Health Sciences (USUHS), National Institutes of Diabetes, Digestive and Kidney Disease (NIDDK), (clinicaltrials.gov identifier NCT00001160) and MedStar Washington Hospital Center Institutional Review Boards, and informed consent was obtained from each patient.

This study consisted of a retrospective analysis of blood samples obtained from patients seen at NIDDK or MedStar Washington Hospital Center for the management of thyroid nodules. All patients underwent surgery (near-total or total thyroidectomy). After surgery, formalin-fixed, paraffin-embedded (FFPE) tissue samples were subjected to Ion Torrent™ Oncomine™ Comensive Assay v3 (OCAv3) next-generation sequencing to determine the final pathology diagnosis and the mutation status of the original tumor. Only the patients with histologically confirmed papillary thyroid cancer (PTC) harboring a *BRAFV600E* mutation (57 patients) were included in this study.

These *BRAFV600E*-positive tumors were further sub-classified into low-, intermediate- and high-risk groups, based upon the criteria of the American Thyroid Association [28]. The low-risk group included intra-thyroidal PTC tumors with complete macroscopic tumor resection, no histological evidence of extra-thyroidal extension or vascular invasion, and no clinically evident lymph node metastases or distant metastases. PTCs that were classified as intermediate-risk tumors demonstrated evidence of microscopic invasion into perithyroidal soft tissue, vascular invasion, or clinical lymph node metastases. High-risk patients had tumors with evidence of distant metastases, macroscopic invasion of the perithyroidal tissue/structures, lymph node metastases $\geq$ 3 cm, or incomplete tumor resection.

2.2. Treatment with RAI, Biochemical Testing and Assessment of Overall Response to Therapy

Radioactive iodine therapy was administered to 46/57 patients. Serum thyroglobulin (Tg) and anti-Tg antibodies (TgAb) levels were measured by the Siemens Immulite 2000 Immunoassay system. The functional sensitivity of this assay was 0.07 ng/mL (Tg), and the lowest reported values were Tg less than 0.2 ng/mL.

The overall response to therapy was evaluated at the last follow-up visit and reported as an excellent response (no evidence of structural disease on imaging, Tg on levothyroxine (LT4) < 0.2 ng/mL and no TgAb); an indeterminate response (nonspecific findings on imaging and/or Tg on LT4 $\geq$ 0.2–< 1 ng/mL or stimulated Tg $\geq$ 1–< 10 ng/mL or stable or declining TgAb titers); a biochemical incomplete response (no evidence of structural disease on imaging and Tg $\geq$ 1 ng/mL on LT4 or stimulated Tg $\geq$ 10 ng/mL or rising TgAb titers); and structural incomplete response (evidence of structural disease on imaging).

2.3. Extraction of Cell Free DNA (cfDNA) from Plasma Samples

Patients underwent a blood draw as part of their treatment evaluation. In total, the blood samples were collected from 57 patients with *BRAFV600E*-positive primary PTCs. Fresh blood (2 mL) samples were drawn into BD Vacutainer EDTA tubes (Cat# 366643), immediately centrifuged at 3000 rpm for 10 min at +4 °C, and the plasma fractions were transferred to a clean tube and re-centrifuged at top speed for another 10 min. The plasma then was then carefully transferred to a clean tube to avoid any possible aspiration of the cell pellet and stored at −80 °C.

The isolation of the cfDNA was performed on the KingFisher™ Duo Prime particle processor (Thermo Fisher Scientific; Waltham, MA, USA) using the MagMax Cell Free DNA isolation kit (Thermo Fisher Scientific; Waltham, MA, USA; cat#A29319). The magnetic bead-based purification format enabled the processing of as little as 600 µL of plasma. For the samples where the plasma volume was less than 600 µL, PBS was added to reach 600 µL and corrected for the dilution factor to obtain a uniform 600 µL cfDNA extraction volume for the whole group. The purified cfDNA sample was eluted in 30 µL volume. The quality of the extracted cfDNA was examined using NanoDrop (Thermo Scientific, Waltham, MA, USA), and the eluates were stored at −80 °C.

2.4. Detection of BRAFV600 Mutation by Digital PCR

Microfluidic digital PCR analyses were performed on a QuantStudio™ 3D Digital PCR System (Life Technologies, Carlsbad, CA, USA) as per the previously published protocol [29]. The rare mutation SNP genotyping assays for *BRAFV600E* (Fluorescein—FAM) which was multiplexed with an assay for the detection of wild-type *BRAF* (2′-chloro-7′phenyl-1,4-dichloro-6-carboxy-fluorescein—VIC) were synthesized by Thermo Fisher Scientific. Reaction mixtures contained 8.75 µL of QuantStudio 3D Digital PCR Master Mix, 0.425 µL of TaqMan Assay by Design primer–probe mix, and a diluted sample of cfDNA. A non-template control of water was run for each assay, as well as positive (BCPAP–*BRAFV600E*-mutant thyroid cancer cell line) and negative (FTC133–*BRAF*-wild-type thyroid cancer cell line) sheared DNA controls. The reaction mixture was loaded onto the Quantstudio 3D digital PCR 20K chip and amplification was performed on the Proflex PCR system under the following conditions: 96 °C for 10 min, 39 cycles at 56 °C for 2 min and at 98 °C for 30 s, followed by a final extension step at 60 °C for 2 min. After amplification, the chips were imaged on the QuantStudio 3D Instrument.

The chips were analyzed by the Quantstudio 3D analysis suite cloud software, which assesses raw data and calculates the estimated concentration of the nucleic acid sequence targeted by the FAM and VIC fluorescent dye-labeled probes according to the Poisson distribution. The thresholds for FAM and VIC detection were manually set based on the results from the no-template control, and a minimum of 15,000 counts was required for analysis. The resulting data were reported in copies/µL together with the results of the data quality assessment metrics. The mutant fraction was calculated with the ratio of FAM counts (*BRAFV600E*) over FAM and VIC counts (*BRAFV600* and *BRAFWT*) and the value standardized as a percentage.

2.5. Improved and Complete Co-Amplification at Lower Denaturation Temperature (ICE-COLD-PCR)

To enhance the sensitivity of the digital PCR method in the detection of *BRAFV600E* mutations, the COLD-PCR application was applied in order to amplify rare mutant copies relative to wild-type (WT). In brief, extracted nucleic acid template (DNA) was combined with a Precipio-manufactured reference sequence (RS). RS is a synthetic, single-stranded, wild-type-specific oligonucleotide reference sequence, which binds to the wild-type template and inhibits its amplification. The oligonucleotide RS contains a 3′-phosphate modification to prevent polymerase extension. The RS is slightly shorter than the length of the PCR amplicon so that it obstructs primer binding and prevents the amplification of wild-type alleles. At a critical denaturation temperature, the RS:WT duplex remains double-stranded, inhibiting the amplification of WT through thermocycling while RS:mutant duplexes are denatured and then exponentially amplified.

COLD-PCR was performed using the *BRAF* exon 15 mutation analysis kit (Precipio, NE, USA) on the Quantstudio Flex system (Thermo Fisher Scientific; Waltham, MA, USA). cfDNA from 25 pg to 1 ng were used as input in a 25 µL PCR mix including RS-oligonucleotide/PCR primer mix, and 2× Polymerase mix. Wild-type and *V600E* controls were also included. An initial denaturation step was performed for 30 s at 98 °C, followed by 45 cycles of ICE-COLD-PCR (10 s of denaturation at 98 °C; 30 s of blocker annealing at 69 °C and 30 s at 74 °C (Tc); 30 s of primer annealing at 63 °C; and 20 s of elongation at 72 °C) to enrich the mutation fraction. An additional five cycles of standard PCR amplification (10 s of denaturation at 98 °C, 10 s of annealing at 63 °C, and 20 s of elongation at 72 °C) was performed with the final extension at 72 °C for 5 min and infinite hold at 12 °C.

Enriched samples were used for the detection of *BRAFV600E* and wild-type *BRAF* alleles by real-time PCR using the Taqman Single-nucleotide polymorphism (SNP) Genotyping assay for *BRAFV600E* (Precipio, NE, USA) or for the detection of *BRAFV600E* and wild-type *BRAF* alleles using microfluidic digital PCR. For real-time PCR, 5 uL of the diluted sample (1 to 200) was added to a master mix containing the 20X Genotyping Assay mix, and the 2× GTXpress master mix. qPCR cycling conditions included an initial denaturation step for 20 s at 95 °C, followed by 40 cycles of 3 s at 95 °C, and 20 s at 60 °C, followed a final cooling step at 4 °C. The TaqMan® Genotyper and real-time PCR instrument software were used for allelic discrimination. Wild-type allele and mutant alleles utilized the VIC and FAM probe, respectively. The genotype assignments were based on the ratio between the fluorescent intensities of VIC and FAM after normalization. A high VIC/FAM ratio represented wild-type alleles and a low VIC/FAM ratio corresponded to mutant alleles. For microfluidic digital PCR, 1 μL of ICE-COLD-PCR product was used and allelic discrimination was performed as described above. Positive control (*BRAFV600-mutant* BCPAP cell line), wild-type (*BRAF* wild-type FTC133 cell line) control and negative template controls (NTC) were included and runs were done in triplicate.

2.6. Statistical Analysis

Data were summarized by using frequencies and percentages for categorical variables and means with standard deviations (SDs) or medians with the 25–75% interquartile range (IQRs) for continuous variables, dependent on the distribution. Shapiro–Wilk's normality test was performed to access normal distribution. Categorical variables were compared between subgroups using the Fisher exact test or the Pearson Chi-square test, when appropriate. Continuous variables were compared with Student's t-test and with the Mann–Whitney test when not following normal distribution. Logistic regression analyses were used to assess if mutation detection was an independent predictor of response to treatment when other clinically relevant predictive variables were kept constant. The odds ratios (OR) were reported along with their 95% confidence intervals (CI). A *p*-value of ≤ 0.05 was considered to be statistically significant in the analyses. Data analysis was performed using IBM SPSS Statistics 25.0 (IBM Corp., Armonk, NY, USA).

3. Results:

3.1. Combination of Microfluidic Digital PCR with COLD-PCR Increases the Sensitivity for Detection of BRAFV600E

We established a protocol to detect *BRAFV600E* in thyroid cancer samples by microfluidic digital PCR and described this technique in a previously published study [29]. In the present study, we applied a similar approach and in addition, used a co-amplification at COLD-PCR prior to digital PCR. Initial experiments were performed using the control DNAs (wild-type *BRAF* and 1% *BRAFV600E*), as well as the DNA extracted from a *BRAFV600E*-positive BCPAP cell line. As demonstrated in Figure 1, COLD-PCR significantly enriched the DNA template in rare mutant copies and increased the sensitivity of digital PCR for the detection of *BRAFV600E* by 100-fold. Subsequently, we used this approach for the analysis of DNA extracted from the plasma samples of patients with thyroid cancer.

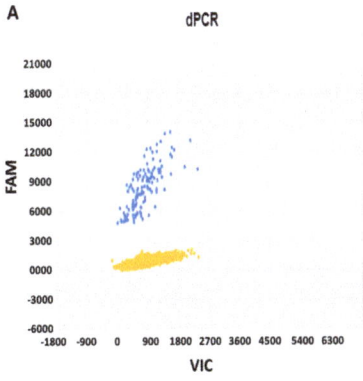

Figure 1. *Cont.*

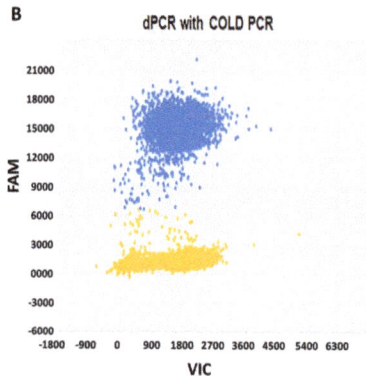

Figure 1. Detection of *BRAFV600E* by microfluidic digital PCR alone or in combination with COLD-PCR. Each panel represents a single experiment whereby DNA from BCPAP cells was segregated into individual wells and assessed for the presence of the mutant alleles using two different fluorophores (FAM and VIC). The signals from the FAM (blue) and VIC (red) dyes are plotted on the Y axis and the X axis, respectively. The yellow cluster represents the unamplified wells (negative calls). (**A**) Two-dimensional plots of microfluidic digital PCR reads out of 1 ng DNA extracted from BCPAP cells. Blue cluster represents the wells that were positive for the *BRAFV600E* mutation. (**B**) Results of dPCR analysis after the enrichment of *BRAFV600E* by COLD-PCR demonstrating 100-fold increase in mutant alleles (blue cluster). dPCR, digital Polymerase chain reaction; COLD, co-amplification at lower denaturation temperature; PCR, Polymerase chain reaction; FAM, fluorescein; VIC, 2′-chloro-7′phenyl-1,4-dichloro-6-carboxy-fluorescein.

3.2. Clinicopathologic Characteristics of BRAFV600E Positive Thyroid Cancers

The study cohort consisted of 57 patients with *BRAFV600E*-positive PTCs, followed for a median of 27 (IQR 16.5–51) months. Of these, 40 (70%) were women, and 17 (30%) were men. The average age of patients was 46 years, ranging from 21 to 82 years. The final pathology revealed a thyroid cancer diagnosis in all patients, including 38 patients with classical PTC (CPTC), 13 with tall cell variant PTC (TCPTC), and six with follicular variant PTC (FVPTC). In one case in addition to CPTC, a micro-medullary thyroid cancer was detected.

The average tumor size was 2.4 ± 1.8 cm, with a multifocal growth pattern found in 34/57 (59.6%) cases and gross extension in 13/57 (22.8%) cases. Lymph node metastases to the central neck and lateral neck compartments were detected in 31/57 (54%) and 18/57 (31%) cases, respectively. Distant metastases were found in 12 patients (in 10 individuals in lungs and two cases in bones). There were 19 patients with low-risk thyroid cancer, 22 patients with intermediate-risk tumors, and in 16 cases the tumors were classified as high-risk PTCs.

3.3. Detection of cfBRAFV600E in Serum from Patients with Low-, Intermediate- and High–Risk PTCs

Microfluidic digital PCR allowed the detection of *cfBRAFV600E* in the DNA extracted from 8/57 (14%) patients. The ratios of the mutant vs. wild-type *BRAF* alleles ranged from 0.6% to 6.9%. By microfluidic dPCR, *cfBRAFV600E* alleles were found in seven patients with high-risk PTCs and one patient with intermediate-risk PTC. The combination of microfluidic dPCR with COLD-PCR allowed the detection of circulating *cfBRAFV600E* in 24/57 (42.1%) examined patients.

Clinicopathological characteristics of the cases in which circulating *cfBRAFV600E* was detected and the cases in which wild-type *BRAF* was detected are summarized and compared in Table 1.

There was no significant correlation between the presence of *cfBRAFV600E* or wild-type *BRAF* in plasma and patient gender and age at diagnosis or histological subtype of tumor. However, the detection of *cfBRAFV600E* was significantly associated with tumor size ($p = 0.03$), multifocal patterns of growth

($p = 0.03$), the presence of extrathyroidal gross extension ($p = 0.02$) and the presence of pulmonary micrometastases ($p = 0.04$).

Table 1. Clinicopathological features of the *BRAFV600*-positive papillary thyroid carcinomas.

Clinical Features	cfBRAFV600E in Plasma (24 Cases)	Wild-Type cfBRAF in Plasma (33 Cases)	p-Value
Age at the time of diagnosis (years)	45.7 ± 16.9	46.5 ± 16.4	0.92
Sex (male/female)	8/16	9/24	0.62
Tumor subtype			
Classical	16 (67%)	22 (67%)	
Follicular variant	2 (8%)	4 (12%)	0.87
Tall cell variant	6 (25%)	7 (21%)	
Tumor size (cm)	2.99 ± 1.9	1.99 ± 1.6	0.03
Multifocal growth	10 (42%)	24 (73%)	0.03
Gross extrathyroidal extension	9 (38%)	4 (12%)	0.02
Lymph node metastasis	16 (67%)	15 (45%)	0.27
Distant metastases	8 (33%)	4 (12%)	0.05
Pulmonary micrometastases	7 (29%)	3 (9%)	0.04

There was no significant correlation between the presence of cfBRAFV600E or wild-type *BRAF* in plasma and patient gender and age at diagnosis or histological subtype of tumor. However, the detection of cfBRAFV600E was significantly associated with tumor size ($p = 0.03$), multifocal patterns of growth ($p = 0.03$), the presence of extrathyroidal gross extension ($p = 0.02$) and the presence of pulmonary micrometastases ($p = 0.04$).

Analysis of cfDNA from blood samples that were obtained in patients with low-, intermediate-, and high-risk PTCs revealed the presence of cfBRAFV600E in 4/19 (21.0%), 8/22 (36.3%) and 12/16 (75.0%) of cases, respectively. The results of the analysis are summarized in Table 2.

Table 2. Risk stratification of the patients with *BRAFV600*-positive papillary thyroid carcinomas.

Risk Stratification	BRAFV600E in Plasma $n = 24$ Cases	Wild-Type BRAF in Plasma $n = 33$ Cases	p-Value
Low risk	4 (21%)	15 (79%)	0.02
Intermediate risk	8 (36%)	14 (64%)	0.48
High risk	12 (75%)	4 (25%)	0.002

In the liquid biopsy from patients with low-risk tumors, cfBRAFV600E alleles were less frequently detected than wild-type *BRAF* ($p = 0.026$). In contrast, in the plasma from the patients with high-risk PTCs, cfBRAFV600E alleles were more frequently detected than wild-type *BRAF* ($p = 0.002$).

3.4. Detection of cfBRAFV600E in Serum Samples and Treatment Outcome

All patients underwent surgery for thyroid cancer. During the follow-up, repeat surgery for metastatic lymph nodes was reported in 12/57 patients, including seven patients with detectable *BRAFV600E* in serum and five patients with circulating wild-type *BRAF*. Treatment with RAI was administered to 46/57 patients (23 with cfBRAFV600E and 23 with wild-type cfBRAF). Multiple treatments with RAI were administered in five patients with cfBRAFV600E and in two patients with wild-type cfBRAF. The median cumulative doses in patients with *BRAFV600E* and wild-type *BRAF* were 145 mci (IQR 250 mci) and 100 mci (IQR 150 mci), respectively, $p = 0.022$.

An overall excellent response was documented in 6/24 (25%) patients with cfBRAFV600E, and in 23/33 (69.6%) patients with wild-type cfBRAF ($p = 0.001$). The analysis of treatment outcomes in patients with low-, intermediate-, and high-risk cancers is presented in Table 3.

A multivariate logistic regression model, including clinically relevant prognostic factors such as age, ATA risk stratification and cfBRAFV600E mutation status, revealed that the detection of cfBRAFV600E was an independent factor for an incomplete response to treatment, along with the baseline pathology associated with a high risk for recurrence. Table 4 shows that the odds of having an incomplete response to treatment is 4.68 times greater for patients with cfBRAFV600E mutation compared to the patients with wild-type *BRAF*, independently of other risk factors (OR, 4.68; 95% CI, 1.26–17.32; $p = 0.02$).

Table 3. Response to the treatment related to risk classification and cfBRAFV600E detection.

Risk Group	# Cases	BRAF Status	# Cases	Excellent Response	Indeterminate Response	Biochemically Incomplete	Structurally Incomplete
Low	19	mutant	4	1	1	2	0
		wild-type	15	14	1	0	0
Intermediate	22	mutant	8	3	3	0	2
		wild-type	14	8	4	0	2
High	16	mutant	12	2	0	4	6
		wild-type	4	1	0	1	2

Table 4. The risk factors associated with non-excellent response to treatment (either biochemical or structurally incomplete or indeterminate response).

Variable	Odds Ratio (OR)	95% Confidence Intervals (CI)		*p* Value
		Lower	Upper	
Age at diagnosis	0.99	0.95	1.04	0.80
cfBRAFV600E detection	4.68	1.26	17.32	0.02
Risk stratification (intermediate vs. low)	2.81	0.62	12.75	0.18
Risk stratification (high vs. low)	9.33	1.539	56.618	0.01

OR, odds ratio; CI, confidence intervals.

3.5. Detection of cfBRAFV600E in Serum Samples from Low-Risk Thyroid Cancer Patients

Low-risk papillary cancers represent the vast majority of thyroid cancers diagnosed today. There is no convincing evidence that aggressive treatment is beneficial for these patients. Therefore, studies that identify molecular markers that would predict the response to treatment in low-risk thyroid cancer patients could be useful.

An association between the presence of cfBRAFV600E and an efficacy of treatment was found when a low-risk group of patients was analyzed. In total, the excellent response to treatment in the low-risk group was documented in 15/19 (78.9%) patients. Among these patients, *BRAFV600E* was detected in the serum in four individuals, and only wild-type *BRAF* was found in 15 patients. An excellent response was reported in 25% (1/4) cases with *BRAFV600E*, and in 93% (14/15) of patients with wild-type *BRAF* ($p = 0.016$).

4. Discussion

Insights into the biological behavior of malignancies were gained by the identification of biomarkers in blood samples, taken at various time points during the course of the disease. Liquid biopsy has been shown to be a viable approach for the minimally-invasive assessment of tumor-specific mutations, and can potentially be used in both clinical and investigational applications [13,14]. Recent studies have demonstrated that liquid biopsy is a useful technique for monitoring the response to treatment in patients with medullary and radioiodine-refractory poorly differentiated thyroid cancers [30,31].

In this study, we examined the utility of liquid biopsy in patients with *BRAFV600E*-mutant PTC. We focused on the detection of cfBRAFV600E, since this is the most frequent genomic alteration found in PTC and a well established druggable target with already approved pharmacological inhibitors of the BRAF/MAPK signaling pathway. We hypothesized that the detection of *BRAFV600E* in liquid biopsy samples from patients with *BRAFV600E*-positive primary PTCs could be correlated with the aggressiveness of thyroid cancer. We also sought to determine the potential utility of this test for the delineation of treatment outcome in patients with PTCs.

The first step was the development of a sensitive assay, capable of detecting low-abundance *BRAFV600E* in the blood samples from patients with thyroid cancer. One approach for the assessment of low-abundance DNA variants involves technologies allowing the preferential enrichment of mutant DNA sequences, such as COLD-PCR [32]. COLD-PCR can be combined with other PCR techniques and evidence indicates that COLD-PCR can be used as a fundamental platform to improve the sensitivity of downstream technologies, including Sanger sequencing, digital PCR and mutation genotyping.

We developed a protocol for the analysis of cf*BRAFV600E*, where microfluidic digital PCR was combined with COLD-PCR. By performing experiments using synthetic DNAs as well as DNA extracted from thyroid cancer cell lines, we demonstrated that the enrichment of mutant alleles using COLD-PCR increases the sensitivity of microfluidic digital PCR by 100-fold, as compared to digital PCR alone. These results suggest that the combination of microfluidic digital PCR with COLD-PCR could be a suitable technique for the assessment of liquid biopsy samples from patients with thyroid cancer.

Then, we applied this approach for the analysis of *BRAFV600E* in DNA extracted from the plasma of patients with PTC. We demonstrated that microfluidic digital PCR allowed the detection of cf*BRAFV600E* in 14% of patients. However, when the enrichment of low-abundance mutations by COLD-PCR was performed prior to dPCR, cf*BRAFV600E* was detected in the blood of 42% of the examined patients. These results show that differences in methodology significantly affect the outcome of the assay, providing an explanation for the conflicting results that have been published. The analysis of *BRAFV600E* in the serum samples from 94 patients with PTC that were performed using real-time PCR demonstrated that none of the patients had a detectable serum *BRAFV600E* mutation [33]. However, another study demonstrated that cf*BRAFV600E* was detected in 20 of 173 PTC patients when the allele-specific real-time PCR method was employed [34]. Methodological differences can also partially account for the unclear association between cf*BRAFV600E* and clinicopathologic characteristics. Thus, while there was no correlation between cf*BRAFV600E* and clinicopathologic data in one study [33], the detection of *BRAFV600E* in the blood was found to be associated with the *BRAF* status in primary tumors and the presence of active disease in another study [34].

In the current study, by using a combination of microfluidic digital PCR and COLD-PCR techniques, we showed that the detection of cf*BRAFV600E* in liquid biopsy has a lower performance as compared to *BRAFV600E* testing in thyroid tissue samples. These results are consistent with the previously published analyses of cf*BRAFV600E* in liquid biopsy samples from patients with thyroid tumors [34–36]. These findings suggest that molecular testing from liquid biopsy samples in patients with thyroid nodules cannot substitute for fine-needle aspiration biopsy.

In patients with thyroid nodules, the detection of *BRAFV600E* in thyroid fine-needle aspiration biopsy is a well established marker of malignancy, and is associated with a greater likelihood of nodal recurrence [5,12]. However, it appears that the *BRAFV600E* mutation alone is of limited value in risk stratification and its detection in fine needle aspiration biopsy (FNAB) samples does not provide definitive information on the degree of tumor aggressiveness, or the presence of extrathyroidal extension or of distant metastases.

In our study, a comparison of two groups of patients (with- and without detectable cf*BRAFV600E* in plasma) revealed that the presence of cf*BRAFV600E* was associated with the size of the primary tumor as well as with the presence of extra-thyroidal gross extension at the time of surgery. In addition, pulmonary micro-metastases were more frequently detected in patients with detectable cf*BRAFV600E*. These observations suggest that in patients with thyroid nodules, the diagnostic workflow might include not only the detection of *BRAFV600E* in FNAB samples, but also the assessment of plasma cf*BRAFV600E*. The combination of a solid and a liquid biopsy could potentially improve the risk stratification in patients with PTC.

The assessment of liquid biopsy samples in patients with low-, intermediate-, and high-risk tumors demonstrated a progressive increase in the frequency of detectable cf*BRAFV600E*. These observations were in agreement with previous reports that have demonstrated an association between the presence of circulating cf*BRAFV600E* and tumor burden in patients with PTC [34,35]. However, in our study, the detection of circulating cfBRAFV600E was not limited to the patients with advanced PTC. Moreover, we demonstrated that the analysis of liquid biopsy can help in the identification of a subset of PTCs with more aggressive characteristics even in the group of low-risk cancer patients. The use of an effective method in the early identification of a thyroid tumor could permit a minimal invasive surgery preventing some of the complication related to conventional surgery [37,38]. Our data suggest the potential utility of liquid biopsy in guiding the surgical decision, however, additional studies addressing this specific question are needed.

Approximately 5% of metastatic thyroid cancer becomes less well differentiated and demonstrates a poor response to treatment [1]. Patients with BRAFV600E-positive thyroid cancer are poor responders or refractory to RAI therapy because this gain-of-function mutation modulates iodine metabolism resulting in a decreased ability of neoplastic cells to uptake and incorporate radioiodine [7,10]. Recently, the FDA approved two small BRAF-specific inhibitors: vemurafenib and dabrafenib for BRAFV600E-positive advanced RAI-refractory thyroid cancer and metastatic PTC. Evidence suggests that BRAF inhibitory agents restore RAI uptake in BRAFV600E iodine-refractory thyroid cancer cells, probably by reactivating the expression of thyroid-specific genes involved in iodine metabolism [39]. In this context, the identification of patients who would benefit from therapy with the pharmacological inhibitors of BRAF is an important issue. In this study, we demonstrated that the detection of cfBRFV600E in liquid biopsy is an independent factor predicting the response to therapy in patients with PTC. Further study could determine whether the evaluation of cfBRFV600E in liquid biopsy samples could identify patients with a risk of incomplete response after RAI treatment who might then be candidates for alternative treatment with BRAF inhibitors.

The utility of liquid biopsy for the monitoring of patients' responses to treatment has been demonstrated in patients with melanoma, colon cancer, and medullary thyroid cancer [13,16,30]. Unfortunately, the design of the current study (retrospective analysis of plasma samples) did not allow for the evaluation of the utility of liquid biopsy for monitoring the response to treatment with RAI over time in the same patients. The only serum marker currently used in the follow-up of PTC is thyroglobulin (Tg), which is extremely sensitive and reliable but may be less informative in some subsets of patients, particularly those with anti-Tg antibodies. The incomplete resection of normal thyroid tissue or the dedifferentiation of thyroid tumors can render the interpretation of thyroglobulin extremely challenging. In such cases, circulating BRAFV600E may provide an additional tool to monitor PTC patients during treatment.

The development of a comprehensive set of molecular variables to improve risk stratification and facilitate the disease follow-up and monitoring of patients' response to treatment is a common trend in cancer research. Results of our study demonstrate that the combination of microfluidic digital PCR with COLD-PCR increases the sensitivity of cfBRAFV600E testing in liquid biopsy samples from patients with papillary thyroid cancer. These results also suggest that the implementation of liquid biopsy in clinical practice can improve risk stratification and the delineation of an optimal therapeutic strategy in patients with PTC.

Author Contributions: Conceptualization—J.K.-G. and V.V.V.; Methodology—K.J., S.T., A.P., M.C.M.-T., J.C., C.J.G.-L., M.W., L.W., K.D.B., A.B., D.Y., V.V.V. and J.K.-G.; Software—D.Y.; Validation—K.J., A.P., M.C.M.-T. and J.C.; Formal analysis—D.Y., J.K.-G. and V.V.V.; Investigation—K.J., S.T., A.P., M.C.M.-T., J.C., C.J.C.-L., M.W., L.W., K.D.B., A.B., D.Y., V.V.V. and J.K.-G.; Resources—J.K.-G. and V.V.V.; Data curation—M.W., D.Y., J.K.-G. and V.V.V.; Writing—K.J., S.T., J.K.-G. and V.V.V.; Writing Review—K.J., S.T., A.P., M.C.M.-T., J.C., C.J.G.-L., M.W., L.W., K.D.B., A.B., D.Y., V.V.V. and J.K.-G.; Visualization—K.J., S.T. and V.V.V.; Supervision—K.D.B., L.W., J.K.-G. and V.V.V.; Project Administration—M.W. and M.C.M.-T.; Funding—J.K.-G. and V.V.V. All authors have read and agreed to the published version of the manuscript.

Funding: This research was funded by the Murtha Cancer Center, grant number PED-86-90-46 and NIDDK grant ZIE DK 04705313.

Acknowledgments: This project was supported in part by The Catherine Heron and Al Schneider Fellowship in Thyroid Cancer. We would like to thank Lee Weinstein for the critical review of the paper. We thank our patients for participation in the study.

Conflicts of Interest: The authors declare no conflict of interest.

Disclaimer: The opinions or assertions contained herein are the private ones of the authors and are not to be construed as official or reflecting the views of the Department of Defense or the Uniformed Services University of the Health Sciences.

References

1. Fagin, J.A.; Wells, S.A., Jr. Biologic and Clinical Perspectives on Thyroid Cancer. *N. Engl. J. Med.* **2016**, *375*, 2307. [CrossRef]
2. Cancer Genome Atlas Research, N. Integrated genomic characterization of papillary thyroid carcinoma. *Cell* **2014**, *159*, 676–690. [CrossRef]
3. Xu, B.; Ibrahimpasic, T.; Wang, L.; Sabra, M.M.; Migliacci, J.C.; Tuttle, R.M.; Ganly, I.; Ghossein, R. Clinicopathologic Features of Fatal Non-Anaplastic Follicular Cell-Derived Thyroid Carcinomas. *Thyroid Off. J. Am. Thyroid Assoc.* **2016**, *26*, 1588–1597. [CrossRef]
4. Landa, I.; Ibrahimpasic, T.; Boucai, L.; Sinha, R.; Knauf, J.A.; Shah, R.H.; Dogan, S.; Ricarte-Filho, J.C.; Krishnamoorthy, G.P.; Xu, B.; et al. Genomic and transcriptomic hallmarks of poorly differentiated and anaplastic thyroid cancers. *J. Clin. Investig.* **2016**, *126*, 1052–1066. [CrossRef]
5. Liu, C.; Chen, T.; Liu, Z. Associations between BRAF(V600E) and prognostic factors and poor outcomes in papillary thyroid carcinoma: A meta-analysis. *World J. Surg. Oncol.* **2016**, *14*, 241. [CrossRef]
6. Xing, M. BRAF V600E mutation and papillary thyroid cancer. *JAMA* **2013**, *310*, 535. [CrossRef]
7. Xing, M.; Westra, W.H.; Tufano, R.P.; Cohen, Y.; Rosenbaum, E.; Rhoden, K.J.; Carson, K.A.; Vasko, V.; Larin, A.; Tallini, G.; et al. BRAF mutation predicts a poorer clinical prognosis for papillary thyroid cancer. *J. Clin. Endocrinol. Metab.* **2005**, *90*, 6373–6379. [CrossRef] [PubMed]
8. Ge, J.; Wang, J.; Wang, H.; Jiang, X.; Liao, Q.; Gong, Q.; Mo, Y.; Li, X.; Li, G.; Xiong, W.; et al. The BRAF V600E mutation is a predictor of the effect of radioiodine therapy in papillary thyroid cancer. *J. Cancer* **2020**, *11*, 932–939. [CrossRef] [PubMed]
9. Wang, F.; Zhao, S.; Shen, X.; Zhu, G.; Liu, R.; Viola, D.; Elisei, R.; Puxeddu, E.; Fugazzola, L.; Colombo, C.; et al. BRAF V600E Confers Male Sex Disease-Specific Mortality Risk in Patients With Papillary Thyroid Cancer. *J. Clin. Oncol. Off. J. Am. Soc. Clin. Oncol.* **2018**, *36*, 2787–2795. [CrossRef] [PubMed]
10. Shen, X.; Zhu, G.; Liu, R.; Viola, D.; Elisei, R.; Puxeddu, E.; Fugazzola, L.; Colombo, C.; Jarzab, B.; Czarniecka, A.; et al. Patient Age-Associated Mortality Risk Is Differentiated by BRAF V600E Status in Papillary Thyroid Cancer. *J. Clin. Oncol. Off. J. Am. Soc. Clin. Oncol.* **2018**, *36*, 438–445. [CrossRef] [PubMed]
11. Zhang, X.; Wang, L.; Wang, J.; Zhao, H.; Wu, J.; Liu, S.; Zhang, L.; Li, Y.; Xing, X. Immunohistochemistry is a feasible method to screen BRAF V600E mutation in colorectal and papillary thyroid carcinoma. *Exp. Mol. Pathol.* **2018**, *105*, 153–159. [CrossRef] [PubMed]
12. Nikiforov, Y.E.; Ohori, N.P.; Hodak, S.P.; Carty, S.E.; LeBeau, S.O.; Ferris, R.L.; Yip, L.; Seethala, R.R.; Tublin, M.E.; Stang, M.T.; et al. Impact of mutational testing on the diagnosis and management of patients with cytologically indeterminate thyroid nodules: A prospective analysis of 1056 FNA samples. *J. Clin. Endocrinol. Metab.* **2011**, *96*, 3390–3397. [CrossRef] [PubMed]
13. Heitzer, E.; Perakis, S.; Geigl, J.B.; Speicher, M.R. The potential of liquid biopsies for the early detection of cancer. *NPJ Precis. Oncol.* **2017**, *1*, 36. [CrossRef] [PubMed]
14. Perakis, S.; Speicher, M.R. Emerging concepts in liquid biopsies. *BMC Med.* **2017**, *15*, 75. [CrossRef]
15. Carow, K.; Read, C.; Hafner, N.; Runnebaum, I.B.; Corner, A.; Durst, M. A comparative study of digital PCR and real-time qPCR for the detection and quantification of HPV mRNA in sentinel lymph nodes of cervical cancer patients. *BMC Res. Notes* **2017**, *10*, 532. [CrossRef]
16. Denis, J.A.; Patroni, A.; Guillerm, E.; Pepin, D.; Benali-Furet, N.; Wechsler, J.; Manceau, G.; Bernard, M.; Coulet, F.; Larsen, A.K.; et al. Droplet digital PCR of circulating tumor cells from colorectal cancer patients can predict KRAS mutations before surgery. *Mol. Oncol.* **2016**, *10*, 1221–1231. [CrossRef]
17. Dong, L.; Wang, S.; Fu, B.; Wang, J. Evaluation of droplet digital PCR and next generation sequencing for characterizing DNA reference material for KRAS mutation detection. *Sci. Rep.* **2018**, *8*, 9650. [CrossRef]
18. Garcia, J.; Dusserre, E.; Cheynet, V.; Bringuier, P.P.; Brengle-Pesce, K.; Wozny, A.S.; Rodriguez-Lafrasse, C.; Freyer, G.; Brevet, M.; Payen, L.; et al. Evaluation of pre-analytical conditions and comparison of the performance of several digital PCR assays for the detection of major EGFR mutations in circulating DNA from non-small cell lung cancers: The CIRCAN_0 study. *Oncotarget* **2017**, *8*, 87980–87996. [CrossRef]

19. Ashida, A.; Sakaizawa, K.; Mikoshiba, A.; Uhara, H.; Okuyama, R. Quantitative analysis of the BRAF V600E mutation in circulating tumor-derived DNA in melanoma patients using competitive allele-specific TaqMan PCR. *Int. J. Clin. Oncol.* **2016**, *21*, 981–988. [CrossRef]
20. Lamy, P.J.; Castan, F.; Lozano, N.; Montelion, C.; Audran, P.; Bibeau, F.; Roques, S.; Montels, F.; Laberenne, A.C. Next-Generation Genotyping by Digital PCR to Detect and Quantify the BRAF V600E Mutation in Melanoma Biopsies. *J. Mol. Diagn.* **2015**, *17*, 366–373. [CrossRef]
21. Li, X.; Liu, Y.; Shi, W.; Xu, H.; Hu, H.; Dong, Z.; Zhu, G.; Sun, Y.; Liu, B.; Gao, H.; et al. Droplet digital PCR improved the EGFR mutation diagnosis with pleural fluid samples in non-small-cell lung cancer patients. *Clin. Chim. Acta Int. J. Clin. Chem.* **2017**, *471*, 177–184. [CrossRef] [PubMed]
22. Sefrioui, D.; Mauger, F.; Leclere, L.; Beaussire, L.; Di Fiore, F.; Deleuze, J.F.; Sarafan-Vasseur, N.; Tost, J. Comparison of the quantification of KRAS mutations by digital PCR and E-ice-COLD-PCR in circulating-cell-free DNA from metastatic colorectal cancer patients. *Clin. Chim. Acta Int. J. Clin. Chem.* **2017**, *465*, 1–4. [CrossRef] [PubMed]
23. Mauger, F.; How-Kit, A.; Tost, J. COLD-PCR Technologies in the Area of Personalized Medicine: Methodology and Applications. *Mol. Diagn. Ther.* **2017**, *21*, 269–283. [CrossRef] [PubMed]
24. Tost, J. The clinical potential of Enhanced-ice-COLD-PCR. *Expert Rev. Mol. Diagn.* **2016**, *16*, 265–268. [CrossRef] [PubMed]
25. Milbury, C.A.; Correll, M.; Quackenbush, J.; Rubio, R.; Makrigiorgos, G.M. COLD-PCR enrichment of rare cancer mutations prior to targeted amplicon resequencing. *Clin. Chem.* **2012**, *58*, 580–589. [CrossRef]
26. Li, J.; Makrigiorgos, G.M. COLD-PCR: A new platform for highly improved mutation detection in cancer and genetic testing. *Biochem. Soc. Trans.* **2009**, *37*, 427–432. [CrossRef]
27. Castellanos-Rizaldos, E.; Milbury, C.A.; Guha, M.; Makrigiorgos, G.M. COLD-PCR enriches low-level variant DNA sequences and increases the sensitivity of genetic testing. *Methods Mol. Biol.* **2014**, *1102*, 623–639. [CrossRef]
28. Haugen, B.R.; Alexander, E.K.; Bible, K.C.; Doherty, G.M.; Mandel, S.J.; Nikiforov, Y.E.; Pacini, F.; Randolph, G.W.; Sawka, A.M.; Schlumberger, M.; et al. 2015 American Thyroid Association Management Guidelines for Adult Patients with Thyroid Nodules and Differentiated Thyroid Cancer: The American Thyroid Association Guidelines Task Force on Thyroid Nodules and Differentiated Thyroid Cancer. *Thyroid Off. J. Am. Thyroid Assoc.* **2016**, *26*, 1–133. [CrossRef]
29. Ylli, D.; Patel, A.; Jensen, K.; Li, Z.Z.; Mendonca-Torres, M.C.; Costello, J.; Gomes-Lima, C.J.; Wartofsky, L.; Burman, K.D.; Vasko, V.V. Microfluidic Droplet Digital PCR Is a Powerful Tool for Detection of BRAF and TERT Mutations in Papillary Thyroid Carcinomas. *Cancers* **2019**, *11*, 1916. [CrossRef]
30. Cote, G.J.; Evers, C.; Hu, M.I.; Grubbs, E.G.; Williams, M.D.; Hai, T.; Duose, D.Y.; Houston, M.R.; Bui, J.H.; Mehrotra, M.; et al. Prognostic Significance of Circulating RET M918T Mutated Tumor DNA in Patients With Advanced Medullary Thyroid Carcinoma. *J. Clin. Endocrinol. Metab.* **2017**, *102*, 3591–3599. [CrossRef]
31. Brose, M.S.; Cabanillas, M.E.; Cohen, E.E.; Wirth, L.J.; Riehl, T.; Yue, H.; Sherman, S.I.; Sherman, E.J. Vemurafenib in patients with BRAF(V600E)-positive metastatic or unresectable papillary thyroid cancer refractory to radioactive iodine: A non-randomised, multicentre, open-label, phase 2 trial. *Lancet Oncol.* **2016**, *17*, 1272–1282. [CrossRef]
32. Fitarelli-Kiehl, M.; Yu, F.; Ashtaputre, R.; Leong, K.W.; Ladas, I.; Supplee, J.; Paweletz, C.; Mitra, D.; Schoenfeld, J.D.; Parangi, S.; et al. Denaturation-Enhanced Droplet Digital PCR for Liquid Biopsies. *Clin. Chem.* **2018**, *64*, 1762–1771. [CrossRef] [PubMed]
33. Kwak, J.Y.; Jeong, J.J.; Kang, S.W.; Park, S.; Choi, J.R.; Park, S.J.; Kim, E.K.; Chung, W.Y. Study of peripheral BRAF(V600E) mutation as a possible novel marker for papillary thyroid carcinomas. *Head Neck* **2013**, *35*, 1630–1633. [CrossRef] [PubMed]
34. Cradic, K.W.; Milosevic, D.; Rosenberg, A.M.; Erickson, L.A.; McIver, B.; Grebe, S.K. Mutant BRAF(T1799A) can be detected in the blood of papillary thyroid carcinoma patients and correlates with disease status. *J. Clin. Endocrinol. Metab.* **2009**, *94*, 5001–5009. [CrossRef] [PubMed]
35. Almubarak, H.; Qassem, E.; Alghofaili, L.; Alzahrani, A.S.; Karakas, B. Non-invasive Molecular Detection of Minimal Residual Disease in Papillary Thyroid Cancer Patients. *Front. Oncol.* **2019**, *9*, 1510. [CrossRef]
36. Li, H.; Zhao, J.; Zhang, J.; Wang, C.; Li, M.; Wu, S.; Su, Z.; Pan, Q. Detection of ctDNA in the plasma of patients with papillary thyroid carcinoma. *Exp. Ther. Med.* **2019**, *18*, 3389–3396. [CrossRef]

37. Calo, P.G.; Medas, F.; Conzo, G.; Podda, F.; Canu, G.L.; Gambardella, C.; Pisano, G.; Erdas, E.; Nicolosi, A. Intraoperative neuromonitoring in thyroid surgery: Is the two-staged thyroidectomy justified? *Int. J. Surg.* **2017**, *41* (Suppl. 1), S13–S20. [CrossRef]
38. Gambardella, C.; Polistena, A.; Sanguinetti, A.; Patrone, R.; Napolitano, S.; Esposito, D.; Testa, D.; Marotta, V.; Faggiano, A.; Calo, P.G.; et al. Unintentional recurrent laryngeal nerve injuries following thyroidectomy: Is it the surgeon who pays the bill? *Int. J. Surg.* **2017**, *41* (Suppl. 1), S55–S59. [CrossRef]
39. Dunn, L.A.; Sherman, E.J.; Baxi, S.S.; Tchekmedyian, V.; Grewal, R.K.; Larson, S.M.; Pentlow, K.S.; Haque, S.; Tuttle, R.M.; Sabra, M.M.; et al. Vemurafenib Redifferentiation of BRAF Mutant, RAI-Refractory Thyroid Cancers. *J. Clin. Endocrinol. Metab.* **2019**, *104*, 1417–1428. [CrossRef]

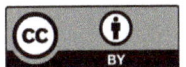

© 2020 by the authors. Licensee MDPI, Basel, Switzerland. This article is an open access article distributed under the terms and conditions of the Creative Commons Attribution (CC BY) license (http://creativecommons.org/licenses/by/4.0/).

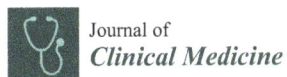

Article

Influence of Care Pathway on Thyroid Nodule Surgery Relevance: A Historical Cohort Study

Solène Castellnou [1],*, Jean-Christophe Lifante [2,3], Stéphanie Polazzi [3,4], Léa Pascal [4], Françoise Borson-Chazot [1,3] and Antoine Duclos [3,4]

[1] Endocrinology Department, Groupement Hospitalier Est, Hospices Civils de Lyon, 69500 Bron, France; francoise.borson-chazot@chu-lyon.fr
[2] Endocrine Surgery Department, Centre Hospitalier Lyon Sud, Hospices Civils de Lyon, 69310 Pierre Bénite, France; jean-christophe.lifante@chu-lyon.fr
[3] Health Services and Performance Research Lab (EA 7425 HESPER), Université Claude Bernard Lyon 1, 69100 Villeurbanne, France; stephanie.polazzi@chu-lyon.fr (S.P.); antoine.duclos@chu-lyon.fr (A.D.)
[4] Health Data Department, Hospices Civils de Lyon, 69003 Lyon, France; lea.pascal@chu-lyon.fr
* Correspondence: solene.castellnou@chu-lyon.fr; Tel.: +33-(0)7-8188-3928

Received: 19 June 2020; Accepted: 15 July 2020; Published: 17 July 2020

Abstract: Background: Guidelines recommend using fine-needle aspiration cytology (FNAC) to guide thyroid nodule surgical indication. However, the extent to which these guidelines are followed remains unclear. This study aimed to analyze the quality of the preoperative care pathway and to evaluate whether compliance with the recommended care pathway influenced the relevance of surgical indications. Methods: Nationwide historical cohort study based on data from a sample (1/97th) of French health insurance beneficiaries. Evaluation of the care pathway of adult patients operated on between 2012 and 2015 during the year preceding thyroid nodule surgery. The pathway containing only FNAC was called "FNAC", the pathway including an endocrinology consultation (ENDO) with FNAC was called "FNAC+ENDO", whereas the no FNAC pathway was called "NO FNAC". The main outcome was the malignant nature of the nodule. Results: Among the 1080 patients included in the study, "FNAC+ENDO" was found in 197 (18.2%), "FNAC" in 207 (19.2%), and "NO FNAC" in 676 (62.6%) patients. Cancer diagnosis was recorded in 72 (36.5%) "FNAC+ENDO" patients and 66 (31.9%) "FNAC" patients, against 119 (17.6%) "NO FNAC" patients. As compared to "NO FNAC", the "FNAC+ENDO" care pathway was associated with thyroid cancer diagnosis (OR 2.67, 1.88–3.81), as was "FNAC" (OR 2.09, 1.46–2.98). Surgeries performed in university hospitals were also associated with thyroid cancer diagnosis (OR 1.61, 1.19–2.17). Increasing the year for surgery was associated with optimal care pathway (2015 vs. 2012, OR 1.52, 1.06–2.18). Conclusions: The recommended care pathway was associated with more relevant surgical indications. While clinical guidelines were insufficiently followed, compliance improved over the years.

Keywords: thyroid nodule; care pathway; guidelines; fine-needle aspiration cytology; thyroid cancer

1. Introduction

The high clinical prevalence of thyroid nodules reaches 5.3–6.4% in women and 0.8–1.3% in men in countries in which iodine intake is sufficient. The prevalence of palpable thyroid nodules increases with age, reaching more than 20% in women after 50 years of age [1–3]. However, their ultrasound (US) prevalence is much higher, reaching more than 60%, and the widespread use of imaging has led to an increase of fortuitous thyroid nodule discoveries over the last years [2,4]. The primary aim of a thyroid nodule investigation is to rule out a malignant tumor. Guidelines recommend performing a Thyroid Stimulating Hormone (TSH) assay for every nodule, as well as a cervical US [5–10]. Depending on both the size and the features of the nodule, fine-needle aspiration cytology

(FNAC) can be required. Cytology results obtained by FNAC determine the need for surgery but are not an automatic indication for surgery [8,11–13]. Surgical indications are standardized and must be restricted to suspicion of malignant, toxic, or compressive nodule. The remaining types of nodules, which are by far more frequent, may be only monitored instead of surgery [14], with active surveillance even being proposed in some instances for papillary thyroid microcarcinoma, a histological type of cancer with low evolutionary potential and very good prognosis [15–17]. Indeed, the increased detection of thyroid nodules has led to an increase in the number of thyroid surgeries, resulting in an overtreatment of thyroid nodules and an excess of avoidable surgeries. Such surgeries can lead to hypothyroidism and complications, such as hypoparathyroidism or recurrent laryngeal nerve paralysis, which are responsible for quality of life deterioration and increased health expenditure [18–21]. The increase in the number of surgeries coupled to the improvement in histology techniques has led to an increase in thyroid cancer incidence over the past 30 years, while thyroid cancer mortality remains low and stable. This fits the definition of overdiagnosis, which involves approximately 70% to 80% of thyroid cancers in France [16,22–28]. Guidelines should allow for better targeting of surgical indications, leading to fewer avoidable surgeries and fewer fortuitous microcancer discoveries. This would have a beneficial effect on patient quality of life, which can be impaired following thyroid surgery or when a thyroid cancer is discovered [29,30]. However, compliance with those guidelines and factors affecting this compliance are difficult to assess. Studies conducted in France in 2010 and in Germany in 2006 found low rates of FNAC prior to thyroid surgery [1,31], while surveys performed in several countries found a heterogeneous management of thyroid nodules [32–34]. Moreover, if some studies suggest that FNAC is the most selective examination for preoperative cancer diagnosis [1,35–37], the impact of this examination on surgery relevance in real practice still needs to be studied.

We hypothesize that better compliance with clinical guidelines and the recommended care pathway for thyroid nodule management is associated with improved adequate surgical indications and a decrease in thyroid surgeries performed for benign nodules. The aims of this study were to assess guideline compliance by studying the quality of the preoperative care pathway, to evaluate whether compliance with the recommended care pathway influences the relevance of surgical indications, and to identify the determinants of compliance with the recommended care pathway.

2. Materials and Methods

2.1. Study Design and Data Source

A historical cohort study was conducted on patients who underwent a surgical procedure for thyroid nodules. Their exposure to care pathways during the 12 months preceding the thyroid surgery was evaluated. Three different types of care pathways were studied. Care pathways were considered optimal when at least a FNAC was performed in accordance with guidelines and non-optimal when no FNAC was performed. In "FNAC+ENDO (endocrinology consultation)" and "FNAC" care pathways a FNAC was performed, however unlike "FNAC", the "FNAC+ENDO" care pathway included an additional consultation with an endocrinologist. "NO FNAC" care pathway was defined by the absence of FNAC.

To retrace the care pathway of in- and out-patients, data were obtained from a general sample of French health insurance beneficiaries (*Echantillon Général des Bénéficiaires*, EGB). The EGB is a permanent representative sample based on a survey at the 97th percentile on the health insurance number of the French nationwide health data system (*Système National des Données de Santé*, SNDS). The SNDS is an exhaustive and anonymous data warehouse that gathers sociodemographic, care reimbursement, and care pathway information regarding both hospital and ambulatory care for the entire French population. Reimbursement information includes medical or paramedical procedures and consultations delivered, as well as medications, presence of a long-term disease, biological sampling, and radiological examination. Those data are matched with hospital care information that pertains International

Classification of Diseases 10 (ICD-10) diagnoses codes and surgical procedures performed in all public and private hospitals.

2.2. Study Population

Adult patients who had a thyroid nodule surgery, including both single nodule and multinodular thyroids (included based on the ICD-10 codes C73, D09.3, D34, D44.0, E01.1, E04.1, and E04.2), between 1 January 2012, and 31 December 2015, in metropolitan France were included in the study. Herein, the index hospital stay refers to the stay during which the thyroid surgery was performed. Patients operated for hyperthyroidism, goiter other than multinodular, or with concurrent parathyroid resection were excluded from the study. In order to consider only patients without medical history of thyroid cancer, patients whose index surgical procedure was a thyroid completion were excluded. Furthermore, when considering the 12 months preceding the index hospital stay, patients in long-term disease treatment for thyroid cancer or who had a thyroid surgery, a cervical lymph node dissection, a radioactive iodine treatment, or a diagnosis of thyroid cancer reported during a hospitalization were also excluded from the study.

2.3. Outcome

The main outcome measure was the nature of the nodule on histopathological analysis. Nodules were considered malignant if a diagnosis of thyroid cancer (ICD-10 codes C73 and D09.3) was recorded during the index hospital stay. Nodules initially considered as benign, whose nature was not specified or uncertain at discharge, were secondarily reclassified as malignant if patients received a radioactive iodine treatment, entered the care pathway for long-term diseases specific to thyroid cancer, were operated for a thyroid completion or for a lymph node dissection, or if a diagnosis of thyroid cancer was recorded during a secondary hospitalization in the 12 months following the surgery date. Patients without cancer diagnosis were divided into 2 categories depending on the ICD-10 codes reported during the index hospital stay: benign nodules (D34, D44.0, E04.1) and multinodular goiter (E01.1, E04.2).

2.4. Statistical Analysis

Continuous variables were reported as the median and range (minimum and maximum), while categorical variables were reported as counts and percentages. For the bivariate analysis, continuous variables were compared between patients with thyroid cancer and the others using Wilcoxon rank-sum test, while categorical variables were compared using Chi-squared test. To evaluate the association between the type of care pathway ("FNAC+ENDO", "FNAC", "NO FNAC") and the probability of having a thyroid cancer, and to identify factors associated with an optimal care pathway, stepwise multivariate logistic regression models were performed, with thyroid cancer (yes vs. no), and optimal care pathway ("FNAC+ENDO" or "FNAC" vs. "NO FNAC") as the dependent variables, respectively. Patient (age, gender, socioeconomic status) and hospital (university hospital or non-university hospital) characteristics, patient area of residency (Paris area or other), and the year of the surgery were considered as covariates. Socio economic status was obtained using data from the Universal Healthcare Coverage (*Couverture Maladie Universelle*, CMU), and we considered being a beneficiary as a marker of precariousness. Indeed, all persons residing in France are covered by the French health insurance system, which includes people who have been living in France on a stable and regular basis for more than 3 months, whose income is below a certain ceiling, and who are entitled to free care through the "Couverture maladie universelle". Restricted cubic splines with 3 knots were used to model the effect of age as a continuous covariate. Explanatory variables were included in the multivariate models at $p < 0.20$ (entry level) and exited by the stepwise procedure at $p \geq 0.10$ (removal level). Two-way interactions were then tested between all variables of the final models with a stepwise procedure (entry level at $p < 0.20$ and removal level at $p \geq 0.05$). Adjusted odds ratios (OR) were presented with their 95% confidence intervals (95% CI). A *p*-value of less than 0.05 was considered to indicate statistical significance. Data manipulation and analyses were performed using SAS software (version 9.4; SAS Institute Inc., Cary, NC, USA).

2.5. Ethical Considerations

This study was strictly observational and based on anonymous data. Therefore, in accordance with the French legislation in place at the time of the study, it did not require the written informed consent of participants or the authorization from an ethics committee. The university hospital of Lyon (*Hospices Civils de Lyon*, HCL), as a health research institute, was authorized to use the EGB database by the National Data Protection Commission (*Commission Nationale de l'Informatique et des Libertés*, CNIL), provided that the researcher followed specific training with certification and recorded their study into the register of EGB studies performed in the institute.

3. Results

A total of 1080 patients who underwent a thyroid nodule surgery between 2012 and 2015 were included in the study (Figure 1).

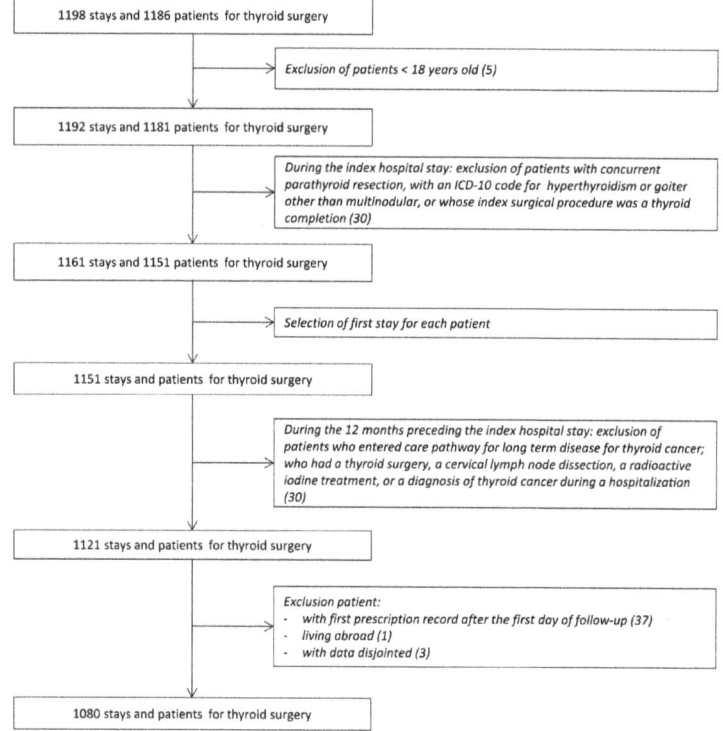

Figure 1. Flow chart.

The majority (77.8%) of patients were females and the median age was 52 years. Overall, a TSH assay was performed in 986 (91.3%) patients, a thyroid US in 906 (83.9%) patients, a FNAC in 404 (37.4%) patients, and a consultation with an endocrinologist in 512 (47.4%) patients. Regarding the type of care pathway, an optimal care pathway was found in 404 (37.4%) patients, with 197 (18.2%) within the "FNAC+ENDO" and 207 (19.2%) within the "FNAC" care pathways, while a non-optimal "NO FNAC" care pathway was found in 676 (62.6%) patients (Figure 2).

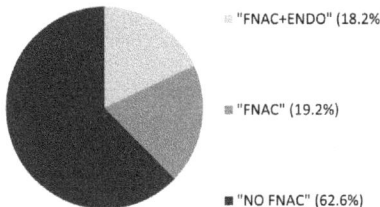

Figure 2. Distribution of the 1080 patients operated on for thyroid nodules between 2012 and 2015 according to the 3 care pathway types. FNAC: Fine-Needle Aspiration Cytology; ENDO: endocrinology consultation.

Surgery was performed in a university hospital for 326 (30.2%) patients. Multinodular goiter was the main reported diagnosis, found in 487 (45.1%) patients, followed by benign nodule in 336 (31.1%) patients, while 257 (23.8%) operated patients were diagnosed with thyroid cancer (Table 1).

Table 1. Characteristics of the 1080 patients who underwent thyroid nodule surgery between 2012 and 2015 according to their distribution in the 3 care pathways.

	Type of Care Pathway before Surgery			Total
	FNAC+ENDO	FNAC	NO FNAC	
Total	197	207	676	1080
Age (years), median (range)	51.0 (18.0–81.0)	51.0 (18.0–85.0)	53.0 (19.0–84.0)	52.0 (18.0–85.0)
Gender				
Male	42 (21.3)	57 (27.5)	141 (20.9)	240 (22.2)
Female	155 (78.7)	150 (72.5)	535 (79.1)	840 (77.8)
Universal healthcare coverage beneficiaries				
Yes	6 (3.0)	13 (6.3)	29 (4.3)	48 (4.4)
No	191 (97)	194 (93.7)	647 (95.7)	1032 (95.6)
Year of surgery				
2012	53 (26.9)	53 (25.6)	202 (29.9)	308 (28.5)
2013	43 (21.8)	47 (22.7)	175 (25.9)	265 (24.5)
2014	53 (26.9)	55 (26.6)	171 (25.3)	279 (25.8)
2015	48 (24.4)	52 (25.1)	128 (18.9)	228 (21.1)
Patient area of residency				
Paris area	41 (20.8)	45 (21.7)	68 (10.1)	154 (14.3)
Other areas	156 (79.2)	162 (78.3)	608 (89.9)	926 (85.7)
Hospital status				
University hospital	61 (31.0)	80 (38.6)	185 (27.4)	326 (30.2)
Non-university hospital public or private	136 (69)	127 (61.4)	491 (72.6)	754 (69.8)
Examinations performed the year before surgery				
TSH assay	188 (95.4)	179 (86.5)	619 (91.6)	986 (91.3)
Cervical US	175 (88.8)	176 (85.0)	555 (82.1)	906 (83.9)
FNAC	197 (100.0)	207 (100.0)	0 (0.0)	404 (37.4)
Endocrinology consultation	197 (100.0)	0 (0.0)	315 (46.6)	512 (47.4)
Type of index thyroid surgery				
Partial	58 (29.4)	88 (42.5)	181 (26.8)	327 (30.3)
Subtotal or total	139 (70.1)	119 (57.5)	495 (73.2)	753 (69.7)
Complementary surgery at 1 year				
Thyroid completion	7 (3.6)	4 (1.9)	12 (1.8)	23 (2.1)
Lymph node dissection (index stay included)	32 (16.2)	26 (12.6)	28 (4.1)	86 (8.0)
Outcomes				
Thyroid pathology				
Cancer	72 (36.5)	66 (31.9)	119 (17.6)	257 (23.8)
Multinodular goiter	66 (33.5)	66 (31.9)	355 (52.5)	487 (45.1)
Benign nodule	59 (29.9)	75 (36.2)	202 (29.9)	336 (31.1)

Data reported as counts (percentages in columns), unless otherwise specified. FNAC: Fine-Needle Aspiration Cytology; ENDO: endocrinology consultation.

In the bivariate analysis, factors associated with a diagnosis of cancer were the type of care pathway and the surgery being performed in a university hospital (both p-value < 0.001). A cancer diagnosis was recorded in 138 (34.2%) patients of the optimal care pathway, including 72 (36.5%) among patients in the "FNAC+ENDO" pathway, and 66 (31.9%) among patients in the "FNAC" pathway, compared with 119 (17.6%) cancer diagnoses for patients in the "NO FNAC" care pathway. In university hospitals, 100 (30.7%) surgeries were associated with a cancer diagnosis, while the same was true for 157 (20.8%) surgeries performed in non-university hospitals (Table 2).

Table 2. Bivariate analysis of factors susceptible to influence thyroid cancer diagnosis among patients operated on for thyroid nodules between 2012 and 2015.

	Malignancy of the Nodule		Total	p-value *
	No	Yes		
Total	823	257	1080	
Type of care pathway				<0.001
FNAC+ENDO	125 (63.5)	72 (36.5)	197	
FNAC	141 (68.1)	66 (31.9)	207	
NO FNAC	557 (82.4)	119 (17.6)	676	
Age (years), median (range)	53.0 (19.0–85.0)	51.0 (18.0–84.0)	52.0 (18.0–85.0)	0.139
Gender				0.175
Male	175 (72.9)	65 (27.1)	240	
Female	648 (77.1)	192 (22.9)	840	
Universal healthcare coverage beneficiaries				0.884
No	786 (76.2)	246 (23.8)	1032	
Yes	37 (77.1)	11 (22.9)	48	
Year of surgery				0.397
2012	237 (76.9)	71 (23.1)	308	
2013	205 (77.4)	60 (22.6)	265	
2014	217 (77.8)	62 (22.2)	279	
2015	164 (71.9)	64 (28.1)	228	
Area of residency of the patient				0.737
Paris area	704 (76.0)	222 (24.0)	926	
Other areas	119 (77.3)	35 (22.7)	154	
Hospital status				<0.001
Non-university hospital, public or private	597 (79.2)	157 (20.8)	754	
University hospital	226 (69.3)	100 (30.7)	326	

Data reported as counts (percentages in lines) unless otherwise specified. * p-values from the Wilcoxon rank-sum test for continuous variables and Chi-squared test for categorical variables. FNAC: Fine-Needle Aspiration Cytology; ENDO: endocrinology consultation.

These associations remained significant in the multivariate analysis. The association of care pathway type with thyroid cancer diagnosis was stronger for "FNAC+ENDO" (OR 2.67; 95% Confidence interval (CI) 1.88–3.81; p-value < 0.001) and "FNAC" (OR 2.09; 95% CI 1.46–2.98; p-value < 0.001) than for "NO FNAC", but the "FNAC+ENDO" care pathway was not significantly more associated with thyroid cancer diagnosis than "FNAC" (OR 1.28; 95% CI 0.85–1.94; p-value = 0.243). Surgeries occurring in university hospitals were significantly associated with thyroid cancer diagnosis (OR 1.61; 95% CI 1.19–2.17; p-value = 0.002; Figure 3) and patients operated on in a university hospital were more susceptible to benefits from the optimal care pathway, with 141 (43.3%) following the recommended care pathway versus 263 (34.9%) in non-university hospitals (OR 1.39; 95% CI 1.06-1.83, p-value = 0.016).

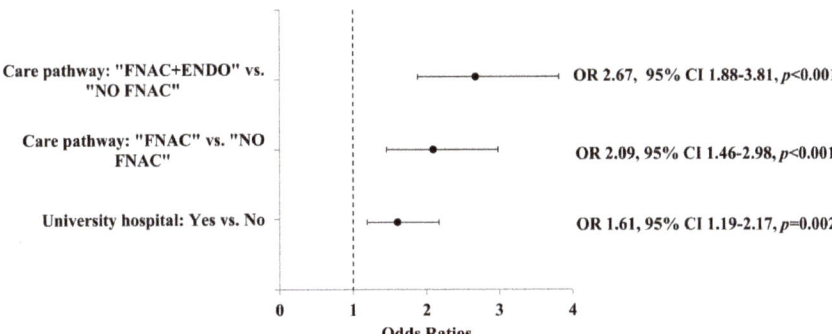

Figure 3. Multivariate analysis of factors having an influence on thyroid cancer diagnosis among patients operated on for thyroid nodules between 2012 and 2015. FNAC: Fine-Needle Aspiration Cytology; ENDO: endocrinology consultation.

Compliance with the recommended care pathway was also associated with patient area of residency, with the likelihood of having an optimal care pathway being higher in the Paris area: 86 (55.8%) patients living in the Paris area had the recommended care pathway versus 318 (34.3%) in other areas (OR 2.43; 95% CI 1.72–3.44, p-value < 0.001). The increase in years for surgery tended to be associated with the optimal care pathway; this association was significant in 2015 vs. 2012 (OR 1.52; 95% CI 1.06–2.18; p-value = 0.021; Figure 4).

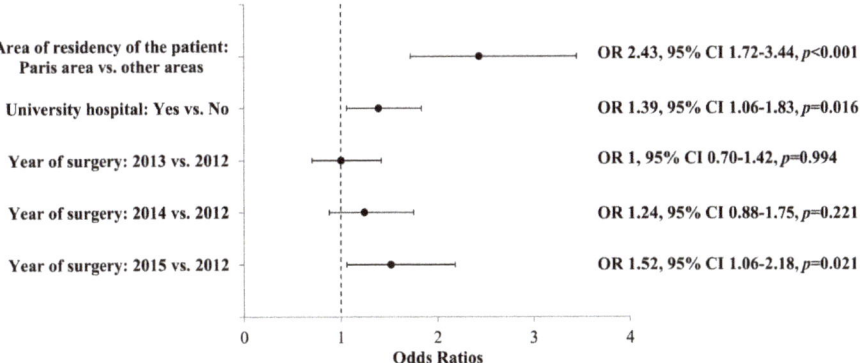

Figure 4. Multivariate analysis of factors having an influence on optimal care pathway compliance among patients operated for thyroid nodule between 2012 and 2015. FNAC: Fine-Needle Aspiration Cytology; ENDO: endocrinology consultation.

4. Discussion

The present population-based study allowed the evaluation in a real-life setting of compliance with guidelines and the association with the relevance of surgical indications for thyroid nodules. Although this study used French data, it is likely that these findings could be generalized, based on the heterogeneity of thyroid nodule management observed in other countries [31–34,38–41]. The majority of surgeries were performed for benign pathology, as approximately only one-quarter were associated with a thyroid cancer diagnosis, suggesting an overtreatment of thyroid nodules. Compliance with guidelines was insufficient, since only one-third of patients in the cohort had a FNAC prior to their thyroid surgery. Herein, compliance with the recommended care pathway was associated with a two-fold increase in the likelihood of performing a surgery for thyroid cancer compared to the non-optimal care pathway. Evaluation of the situation and requirement for surgery might be improved if an endocrinology consultation is proposed, as the "FNAC+ENDO" care pathway was found to be more associated with cancer diagnosis than "FNAC", although not significantly.

The quality and safety of care are at the heart of current priorities. It is mandatory to reduce the number of non-necessary surgeries, can lead to hypothyroidism, and therefore the need for life-long thyroid hormone supplementation, and which are responsible for complications. All this reduces the quality of life of patients and results in medical costs [42]. The discovery of an incidental thyroid cancer, even one with an excellent prognosis such as micropapillary thyroid cancer, can be stressful for the patient, who will require life-long follow-up. In addition, it can have financial consequences for the patient, as a loan may be more difficult to obtain after a cancer diagnosis. FNAC is recommended in all guidelines [7–10,43] to help select patients requiring surgery, since studies have reported FNAC to be the most useful tool for preoperative diagnosis of thyroid cancer [1,35–38]. One of the advantages of the present study is that it allowed the evaluation of guideline compliance and the resulting outcome in real practice, in a nationwide historical cohort study, and on patients managed in or outside hospitals. The results herein confirm that guideline compliance improves surgical indication relevance; however, guideline observance is far from systematic. Regional disparities have previously been observed [1] and seem to persist, as highlighted by the fact that the Paris area was more associated with an optimal care pathway than other areas. This could be partly explained by the high medical density and better access to continuous medical education of the Paris area [44]. Surgeries performed in university hospitals were associated with better compliance with the optimal care pathway, potentially highlighting the increased thyroid cancer diagnosis associated with these hospitals. It is, however, important to bear in mind that university hospitals also have a higher recruitment of cancer patients and might be better trained for selection of surgical indication. Differences in thyroid nodule management are also probably due to an inadequate dissemination of information. Guidelines need to be communicated to all actors involved in thyroid pathologies. Various health professionals, such as surgeons or general practitioners, practicing either outside or inside hospitals are involved and need to be trained in order to improve the quality of care pathways and to homogenize thyroid nodule management within the country.

We chose to conduct this study using the EGB, a representative sample of the French population covered by the national health insurance, obtained from the SNDS. Data about medical resource utilization and both hospital and ambulatory care are prospectively collected in an exhaustive way into this rich database, giving access to real-world data. However, although data from the SNDS give access to reimbursement information, the results of examinations, clinical data, as well as the medical history of patients are not precisely available. Since FNAC results were not known, it was not possible to assess whether the surgical indication when a FNAC was performed was truly based on the obtained cytological result. We chose to include patients with multinodular goiter in the study, as multiple thyroid nodules are quite frequent and because suspicious nodules in multinodular goiter are not an uncommon cause for surgery. However, for a certain proportion of patients, surgical indication could have been retained due to symptomatic or progressive goiter. This is probably the case for a certain number of patients in the "NO FNAC" care pathway, as the proportion of patients with multinodular goiter was more important in this group. This indicates that not all surgeries for benign disease are avoidable. Furthermore, a certain proportion of thyroid cancer in the cohort might have been related to fortuitous discoveries, although this is difficult to assess, since symptoms and pathology analysis were unknown [45,46]. A previous study showed that incidental cancer discovery was more common in multinodular goiter than in thyroid operations for a nodule [35]. Therefore, we can assume that the proportion of fortuitous cancer findings was higher in the non-optimal care pathway groups, with the proportion of goiters being higher in this group. Less than one-fifth of patients had both a FNAC and an endocrinology consultation. This could be explained by the fact that in some cases, such as patients undergoing surgery for progressive nodules after several years of follow-up, a FNAC might have been performed initially but would not be repeated before surgery. This could also explain the proportion of patients who did not have FNAC prior to the operation even though they were under the care of an endocrinologist.

FNAC must be performed according to well defined indications, when the size and characteristics of the nodule upon US examination require it [10,13]. All care pathways with FNAC were considered optimal because the size and features of the nodule were not known. It has been reported that more than half of FNAC are unnecessary [47]. Therefore, US needs to be performed by trained radiologists with thyroid expertise to improve pre-operative assessment of thyroid nodules and better assess the need for FNAC, as unnecessary FNAC can lead to diagnosis difficulties and avoidable surgeries. Moreover, FNAC has a high sensitivity for thyroid cancer diagnosis, at around 94–97%, but a poor specificity and positive predictive value, with both estimated to be approximately 50% [13,48]. This could partly explain the low thyroid cancer prevalence (30 to 40%) often observed among operated patients who have had a FNAC prior to surgery [13,36,48–50], a result concordant with the result observed herein. This low prevalence also likely reflects the heterogeneity of patients undergoing surgery, as some will be operated on for other reasons than a suspicious malignant nodule. Moreover, cytological analysis needs to be performed by an expert pathologist and the addition of molecular analysis in some cases could also help improve accuracy during optimal care pathway diagnosis. Results should be discussed and coordination between general practitioners, specialists, hospital care, and ambulatory care should be developed in order to help decision-making and enhance surgical indication relevance. The management of thyroid nodules of indeterminate risk of malignancy needs to be more standardized. When possible, and after taking into account the preferences of informed patients, more conservative approaches than surgery should be encouraged. Patient willingness to be operated on or not is indeed an important factor to consider. Informing patients about their pathology and reassuring them in cases of benign nodules is essential to promote shared decision-making and is probably one of the key factors to decrease the number of thyroid surgeries.

Even if there is room for progress, the present results found an improvement in optimal care pathway compliance over time, suggestive of an increase in guideline dissemination. Further studies are needed to understand all factors affecting guideline knowledge and compliance and to establish useful actions to improve these.

5. Conclusions

The proportion of thyroid surgery performed for benign nodules is excessively high. This highlights the need to improve risk stratification for better surgical indications. The care pathway recommended in current guidelines is effective in decreasing avoidable surgeries but is insufficiently followed, although improvements have been observed over the years. Interventions are necessary to improve current practice and address geographical disparities.

Author Contributions: Conceptualization, S.C., J.-C.L., F.B.-C., and A.D.; methodology, S.P., L.P., and A.D.; software S.P. and L.P.; validation, A.D., J.-C.L., and F.B.-C.; formal analysis, S.P. and L.P.; investigation, J.-C.L. and F.B.-C.; resources, A.D.; data curation, S.P. and L.P.; writing—original draft preparation, S.C. and A.D.; writing—review and editing, S.C., J.-C.L., S.P., L.P., F.B.-C., and A.D.; visualization, S.C., S.P., and L.P.; supervision, A.D., J.-C.L., and F.B.-C.; project administration, A.D. All authors have read and agreed to the published version of the manuscript.

Funding: This research did not receive any specific grant from any funding agency in the public, commercial, or not-for-profit sector.

Acknowledgments: We thank Véréna Landel for help in manuscript preparation.

Conflicts of Interest: The authors declare no conflict of interest.

References

1. Mathonnet, M.; Cuerq, A.; Tresallet, C.; Thalabard, J.-C.; Fery-Lemonnier, E.; Russ, G.; Leenhardt, L.; Bigorgne, C.; Tuppin, P.; Millat, B.; et al. What is the care pathway of patients who undergo thyroid surgery in France and its potential pitfalls? A national cohort. *BMJ Open* **2017**, *7*, e013589. [CrossRef] [PubMed]

2. Russ, G.; Leboulleux, S.; Leenhardt, L.; Hegedüs, L. Thyroid incidentalomas: Epidemiology, risk stratification with ultrasound and workup. *Eur. Thyroid J.* **2014**, *3*, 154–163. [CrossRef] [PubMed]
3. Valeix, P.; Zarebska, M.; Bensimon, M.; Cousty, C.; Bertrais, S.; Galan, P.; Hercberg, S. Ultrasonic assessment of thyroid nodules, and iodine status of French adults participating in the SU.VI.MAX study. *Ann. Endocrinol.* **2001**, *62*, 499–506.
4. Guth, S.; Theune, U.; Aberle, J.; Galach, A.; Bamberger, C.M. Very high prevalence of thyroid nodules detected by high frequency (13 MHz) ultrasound examination. *Eur. J. Clin. Investig.* **2009**, *39*, 699–706. [CrossRef] [PubMed]
5. Burman, K.D.; Wartofsky, L. CLINICAL PRACTICE. Thyroid Nodules. *N. Engl. J. Med.* **2015**, *373*, 2347–2356. [CrossRef]
6. Brito, J.P.; Yarur, A.J.; Prokop, L.J.; McIver, B.; Murad, M.H.; Montori, V.M. Prevalence of thyroid cancer in multinodular goiter versus single nodule: A systematic review and meta-analysis. *Thyroid Off. J. Am. Thyroid Assoc.* **2013**, *23*, 449–455. [CrossRef]
7. Haugen, B.R.; Alexander, E.K.; Bible, K.C.; Doherty, G.M.; Mandel, S.J.; Nikiforov, Y.E.; Pacini, F.; Randolph, G.W.; Sawka, A.M.; Schlumberger, M.; et al. 2015 American Thyroid Association Management Guidelines for Adult Patients with Thyroid Nodules and Differentiated Thyroid Cancer: The American Thyroid Association Guidelines Task Force on Thyroid Nodules and Differentiated Thyroid Cancer. *Thyroid* **2016**, *26*, 1–133. [CrossRef]
8. Russ, G.; Bonnema, S.J.; Erdogan, M.F.; Durante, C.; Ngu, R.; Leenhardt, L. European Thyroid Association Guidelines for Ultrasound Malignancy Risk Stratification of Thyroid Nodules in Adults: The EU-TIRADS. *Eur. Thyroid J.* **2017**, *6*, 225–237. [CrossRef]
9. Wémeau, J.-L.; Sadoul, J.-L.; d'Herbomez, M.; Monpeyssen, H.; Tramalloni, J.; Leteurtre, E.; Borson-Chazot, F.; Caron, P.; Carnaille, B.; Léger, J.; et al. Guidelines of the French society of endocrinology for the management of thyroid nodules. *Ann. Endocrinol.* **2011**, *72*, 251–281. [CrossRef]
10. American Thyroid Association (ATA) Guidelines Taskforce on Thyroid Nodules and Differentiated Thyroid Cancer; Cooper, D.S.; Doherty, G.M.; Haugen, B.R.; Hauger, B.R.; Kloos, R.T.; Lee, S.L.; Mandel, S.J.; Mazzaferri, E.L.; McIver, B.; et al. Revised American Thyroid Association management guidelines for patients with thyroid nodules and differentiated thyroid cancer. *Thyroid Off. J. Am. Thyroid Assoc.* **2009**, *19*, 1167–1214. [CrossRef]
11. Maino, F.; Forleo, R.; Martinelli, M.; Fralassi, N.; Barbato, F.; Pilli, T.; Capezzone, M.; Brilli, L.; Ciuoli, C.; Di Cairano, G.; et al. Prospective Validation of ATA and ETA Sonographic Pattern Risk of Thyroid Nodules Selected for FNAC. *J. Clin. Endocrinol. Metab.* **2018**, *103*, 2362–2368. [CrossRef]
12. Cibas, E.S.; Ali, S.Z. The 2017 Bethesda System for Reporting Thyroid Cytopathology. *Thyroid Off. J. Am. Thyroid Assoc.* **2017**, *27*, 1341–1346. [CrossRef]
13. Bongiovanni, M.; Spitale, A.; Faquin, W.C.; Mazzucchelli, L.; Baloch, Z.W. The Bethesda System for Reporting Thyroid Cytopathology: A meta-analysis. *Acta Cytol.* **2012**, *56*, 333–339. [CrossRef]
14. Durante, C.; Grani, G.; Lamartina, L.; Filetti, S.; Mandel, S.J.; Cooper, D.S. The Diagnosis and Management of Thyroid Nodules: A Review. *JAMA* **2018**, *319*, 914–924. [CrossRef]
15. Ito, Y.; Miyauchi, A.; Inoue, H.; Fukushima, M.; Kihara, M.; Higashiyama, T.; Tomoda, C.; Takamura, Y.; Kobayashi, K.; Miya, A. An observational trial for papillary thyroid microcarcinoma in Japanese patients. *World J. Surg.* **2010**, *34*, 28–35. [CrossRef]
16. Leboulleux, S.; Tuttle, R.M.; Pacini, F.; Schlumberger, M. Papillary thyroid microcarcinoma: Time to shift from surgery to active surveillance? *Lancet Diabetes Endocrinol.* **2016**, *4*, 933–942. [CrossRef]
17. Filetti, S.; Durante, C.; Hartl, D.; Leboulleux, S.; Locati, L.D.; Newbold, K.; Papotti, M.G.; Berruti, A.; ESMO Guidelines Committee. Electronic address: Clinicalguidelines@esmo.org Thyroid cancer: ESMO Clinical Practice Guidelines for diagnosis, treatment and follow-up. *Ann. Oncol. Off. J. Eur. Soc. Med. Oncol.* **2019**, *30*, 1856–1883. [CrossRef] [PubMed]
18. Lifante, J.-C.; Payet, C.; Ménégaux, F.; Sebag, F.; Kraimps, J.-L.; Peix, J.-L.; Pattou, F.; Colin, C.; Duclos, A. CATHY Study Group Can we consider immediate complications after thyroidectomy as a quality metric of operation? *Surgery* **2017**, *161*, 156–165. [CrossRef] [PubMed]
19. Weiss, A.; Lee, K.C.; Brumund, K.T.; Chang, D.C.; Bouvet, M. Risk factors for hematoma after thyroidectomy: Results from the nationwide inpatient sample. *Surgery* **2014**, *156*, 399–404. [CrossRef] [PubMed]

20. Duclos, A.; Peix, J.-L.; Colin, C.; Kraimps, J.-L.; Menegaux, F.; Pattou, F.; Sebag, F.; Touzet, S.; Bourdy, S.; Voirin, N.; et al. Influence of experience on performance of individual surgeons in thyroid surgery: Prospective cross sectional multicentre study. *BMJ* **2012**, *344*, d8041. [CrossRef] [PubMed]
21. Brito, J.P.; Morris, J.C.; Montori, V.M. Thyroid cancer: Zealous imaging has increased detection and treatment of low risk tumours. *BMJ* **2013**, *347*, f4706. [CrossRef] [PubMed]
22. Vaccarella, S.; Franceschi, S.; Bray, F.; Wild, C.P.; Plummer, M.; Dal Maso, L. Worldwide Thyroid-Cancer Epidemic? The Increasing Impact of Overdiagnosis. *N. Engl. J. Med.* **2016**, *375*, 614–617. [CrossRef] [PubMed]
23. Vaccarella, S.; Dal Maso, L.; Laversanne, M.; Bray, F.; Plummer, M.; Franceschi, S. The Impact of Diagnostic Changes on the Rise in Thyroid Cancer Incidence: A Population-Based Study in Selected High-Resource Countries. *Thyroid Off. J. Am. Thyroid Assoc.* **2015**, *25*, 1127–1136. [CrossRef]
24. Esserman, L.J.; Thompson, I.M.; Reid, B.; Nelson, P.; Ransohoff, D.F.; Welch, H.G.; Hwang, S.; Berry, D.A.; Kinzler, K.W.; Black, W.C.; et al. Addressing overdiagnosis and overtreatment in cancer: A prescription for change. *Lancet Oncol.* **2014**, *15*, e234–e242. [CrossRef]
25. Jegerlehner, S.; Bulliard, J.-L.; Aujesky, D.; Rodondi, N.; Germann, S.; Konzelmann, I.; Chiolero, A. NICER Working Group Overdiagnosis and overtreatment of thyroid cancer: A population-based temporal trend study. *PLoS ONE* **2017**, *12*, e0179387. [CrossRef] [PubMed]
26. Colonna, M.; Uhry, Z.; Guizard, A.V.; Delafosse, P.; Schvartz, C.; Belot, A.; Grosclaude, P. FRANCIM network Recent trends in incidence, geographical distribution, and survival of papillary thyroid cancer in France. *Cancer Epidemiol.* **2015**, *39*, 511–518. [CrossRef]
27. Wiltshire, J.J.; Drake, T.M.; Uttley, L.; Balasubramanian, S.P. Systematic Review of Trends in the Incidence Rates of Thyroid Cancer. *Thyroid Off. J. Am. Thyroid Assoc.* **2016**, *26*, 1541–1552. [CrossRef]
28. Miyauchi, A.; Ito, Y.; Oda, H. Insights into the Management of Papillary Microcarcinoma of the Thyroid. *Thyroid Off. J. Am. Thyroid Assoc.* **2018**, *28*, 23–31. [CrossRef]
29. Roth, E.M.; Lubitz, C.C.; Swan, J.S.; James, B.C. Patient-Reported Quality-of-Life Outcome Measures in the Thyroid Cancer Population. *Thyroid Off. J. Am. Thyroid Assoc.* **2020**. [CrossRef]
30. Singer, S.; Lincke, T.; Gamper, E.; Bhaskaran, K.; Schreiber, S.; Hinz, A.; Schulte, T. Quality of life in patients with thyroid cancer compared with the general population. *Thyroid Off. J. Am. Thyroid Assoc.* **2012**, *22*, 117–124. [CrossRef]
31. Wienhold, R.; Scholz, M.; Adler, J.R.-B.; G Nster, C.; Paschke, R. The management of thyroid nodules: A retrospective analysis of health insurance data. *Dtsch. Arzteblatt Int.* **2013**, *110*, 827–834. [CrossRef]
32. Burch, H.B.; Burman, K.D.; Cooper, D.S.; Hennessey, J.V.; Vietor, N.O. A 2015 Survey of Clinical Practice Patterns in the Management of Thyroid Nodules. *J. Clin. Endocrinol. Metab.* **2016**, *101*, 2853–2862. [CrossRef]
33. Isik, A.; Firat, D.; Yilmaz, I.; Peker, K.; Idiz, O.; Yilmaz, B.; Demiryilmaz, I.; Celebi, F. A survey of current approaches to thyroid nodules and thyroid operations. *Int. J. Surg. Lond. Engl.* **2018**, *54*, 100–104. [CrossRef]
34. Walsh, J.P.; Ryan, S.A.; Lisewski, D.; Alhamoudi, M.Z.; Brown, S.; Bennedbaek, F.N.; Hegedüs, L. Differences between endocrinologists and endocrine surgeons in management of the solitary thyroid nodule. *Clin. Endocrinol. (Oxf.)* **2007**, *66*, 844–853. [CrossRef]
35. Hafdi-Nejjari, Z.; Abbas-Chorfa, F.; Decaussin-Petrucci, M.; Berger, N.; Couray-Targe, S.; Schott, A.-M.; Sturm, N.; Dumollard, J.M.; Roux, J.J.; Beschet, I.; et al. Impact of thyroid surgery volume and pathologic detection on risk of thyroid cancer: A geographical analysis in the Rhône-Alpes region of France. *Clin. Endocrinol. (Oxf.)* **2018**, *89*, 824–833. [CrossRef]
36. Rabal Fueyo, A.; Vilanova Serra, M.; Lerma Puertas, E.; Montserrat Esplugas, E.; Pérez García, J.I.; Mato Matute, E.; De Leiva Hidalgo, A.; Moral Duarte, A. Diagnostic accuracy of ultrasound and fine-needle aspiration in the study of thyroid nodule and multinodular goitre. *Endocrinol. Diabetes Metab.* **2018**, *1*, e00024. [CrossRef]
37. Muratli, A.; Erdogan, N.; Sevim, S.; Unal, I.; Akyuz, S. Diagnostic efficacy and importance of fine-needle aspiration cytology of thyroid nodules. *J. Cytol.* **2014**, *31*, 73–78. [CrossRef] [PubMed]
38. Reinisch, A.; Malkomes, P.; Habbe, N.; Bojunga, J.; Grünwald, F.; Badenhoop, K.; Bechstein, W.O.; Holzer, K. Guideline Compliance in Surgery for Thyroid Nodules—A Retrospective Study. *Exp. Clin. Endocrinol. Diabetes Off. J. Ger. Soc. Endocrinol. Ger. Diabetes Assoc.* **2017**, *125*, 327–334. [CrossRef]

39. Adam, M.A.; Goffredo, P.; Youngwirth, L.; Scheri, R.P.; Roman, S.A.; Sosa, J.A. Same thyroid cancer, different national practice guidelines: When discordant American Thyroid Association and National Comprehensive Cancer Network surgery recommendations are associated with compromised patient outcome. *Surgery* **2016**, *159*, 41–50. [CrossRef]
40. Famakinwa, O.M.; Roman, S.A.; Wang, T.S.; Sosa, J.A. ATA practice guidelines for the treatment of differentiated thyroid cancer: Were they followed in the United States? *Am. J. Surg.* **2010**, *199*, 189–198. [CrossRef]
41. Zolin, S.J.; Burneikis, T.; Rudin, A.V.; Shirley, R.B.; Siperstein, A. Analysis of a thyroid nodule care pathway: Opportunity to improve compliance and value of care. *Surgery* **2019**, *166*, 691–697. [CrossRef]
42. Daher, R.; Lifante, J.-C.; Voirin, N.; Peix, J.-L.; Colin, C.; Kraimps, J.-L.; Menegaux, F.; Pattou, F.; Sebag, F.; Touzet, S.; et al. Is it possible to limit the risks of thyroid surgery? *Ann. Endocrinol.* **2015**, *76*, 1S16-26. [CrossRef]
43. Perros, P.; Boelaert, K.; Colley, S.; Evans, C.; Evans, R.M.; Gerrard Ba, G.; Gilbert, J.; Harrison, B.; Johnson, S.J.; Giles, T.E.; et al. Guidelines for the management of thyroid cancer. *Clin. Endocrinol. (Oxf.)* **2014**, *81* (Suppl. 1), 1–122. [CrossRef]
44. Données de Cadrage: Démographie et Activité des Professions de Santé: Démographie des Médecins—IRDES. Available online: https://www.irdes.fr/EspaceEnseignement/ChiffresGraphiques/Cadrage/DemographieProfSante/DemoMedecins.htm (accessed on 23 October 2019).
45. Ahn, H.S.; Kim, H.J.; Welch, H.G. Korea's thyroid-cancer "epidemic"—Screening and overdiagnosis. *N. Engl. J. Med.* **2014**, *371*, 1765–1767. [CrossRef]
46. Ahn, H.S.; Welch, H.G. South Korea's Thyroid-Cancer "Epidemic"—Turning the Tide. *N. Engl. J. Med.* **2015**, *373*, 2389–2390. [CrossRef]
47. Grani, G.; Lamartina, L.; Ascoli, V.; Bosco, D.; Biffoni, M.; Giacomelli, L.; Maranghi, M.; Falcone, R.; Ramundo, V.; Cantisani, V.; et al. Reducing the Number of Unnecessary Thyroid Biopsies While Improving Diagnostic Accuracy: Toward the "Right" TIRADS. *J. Clin. Endocrinol. Metab.* **2019**, *104*, 95–102. [CrossRef]
48. Ronen, O.; Cohen, H.; Abu, M. Review of a single institution's fine needle aspiration results for thyroid nodules: Initial observations and lessons for the future. *Cytopathol. Off. J. Br. Soc. Clin. Cytol.* **2019**. [CrossRef]
49. Lasolle, H.; Riche, B.; Decaussin-Petrucci, M.; Dantony, E.; Lapras, V.; Cornu, C.; Lachuer, J.; Peix, J.-L.; Lifante, J.-C.; Capraru, O.-M.; et al. Predicting thyroid nodule malignancy at several prevalence values with a combined Bethesda-molecular test. *Transl. Res. J. Lab. Clin. Med.* **2017**, *188*, 58–66.e1. [CrossRef]
50. Jo, V.Y.; Stelow, E.B.; Dustin, S.M.; Hanley, K.Z. Malignancy risk for fine-needle aspiration of thyroid lesions according to the Bethesda System for Reporting Thyroid Cytopathology. *Am. J. Clin. Pathol.* **2010**, *134*, 450–456. [CrossRef] [PubMed]

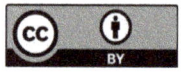

© 2020 by the authors. Licensee MDPI, Basel, Switzerland. This article is an open access article distributed under the terms and conditions of the Creative Commons Attribution (CC BY) license (http://creativecommons.org/licenses/by/4.0/).

MDPI
St. Alban-Anlage 66
4052 Basel
Switzerland
Tel. +41 61 683 77 34
Fax +41 61 302 89 18
www.mdpi.com

Journal of Clinical Medicine Editorial Office
E-mail: jcm@mdpi.com
www.mdpi.com/journal/jcm

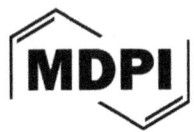

www.ingramcontent.com/pod-product-compliance
Lightning Source LLC
LaVergne TN
LVHW070610100526
838202LV00012B/609